Praise for *When Nurses Hurt Nurses: Recognizing and Overcoming the Cycle of Nurse Bullying*

"If bullying among nurses bewilders you, this book is the key to unlock those obscurities. I recommend this book to every nurse who has experienced, observed, or has questions about workplace bullying. This work should certainly be required reading for anyone who is serious about creating a safer, more respectful workplace."

—Carol F. Rocker, MHS, BN, RN
Vancouver Island Health Authority and Alberta Health Services
Duncan, British Columbia, Canada

"You don't have to look far to find something in the news about bullying. But, you may ask, bullying in nursing? Unfortunately, the answer is 'YES!' While the statistics highlighted in When Nurses Hurt Nurses: Overcoming the Cycle of Nurse Bullying *may be overwhelming, they are not surprising. Cheryl Dellasega has provided insight on this destructive behavior that nursing has perpetuated for far too long. Kudos to Dellasega for lifting the veil that covers this type of negative conduct and opening the door to understanding and addressing bullying in nursing practice."*

—Jan Cooper, PhD, RN
Assistant Professor
University of Mississippi Medical Center School of Nursing
Clinical Simulation Center Director
Vicksburg, Mississippi, USA

When Nurses Hurt Nurses

Recognizing and Overcoming
the Cycle of Nurse Bullying

Cheryl Dellasega, PhD, CRNP

Sigma Theta Tau International
Honor Society of Nursing®

Sigma Theta Tau International

> The Honor Society of Nursing, Sigma Theta Tau International, the only international honor society worldwide, is a global community of nurse leaders with members who live in 86 countries and belong to 469 chapters. Through this network, members lead in using knowledge, scholarship, service, and learning to improve the health of the world's people.

Sigma Theta Tau International
550 West North Street
Indianapolis, IN 46202

To order additional books, buy in bulk, or order for corporate use, contact Nursing Knowledge International at TOLL FREE: +1.888.654.4968 (US / Canada) or +1.317.634.8171 (outside US and Canada).

To request a review copy for course adoption, e-mail solutions@nursingknowledge.org or call TOLL FREE: +1.888.654.4968 (US / Canada) or +1.317.634.8171 (outside US and Canada).

To request author information, or for speaker or other media requests, contact Rachael McLaughlin of the Honor Society of Nursing, Sigma Theta Tau International at 888.634.7575 (US and Canada) or +1.317.634.8171 (outside US and Canada).

ISBN-13: 978-1-935476-56-6

Library of Congress Cataloging-in-Publication Data

Dellasega, Cheryl.
  When nurses hurt nurses : recognizing and overcoming the cycle of nurse bullying / Cheryl Dellasega.
    p. ; cm.
  Includes bibliographical references.
  ISBN 978-1-935476-56-6 (alk. paper)
  1. Nurses--Psychology. 2. Interprofessional relations. 3. Bullying in the workplace. I. Sigma Theta Tau International. II. Title.
  [DNLM: 1. Nurses--psychology. 2. Bullying. 3. Interprofessional Relations. 4. Workplace--psychology. WY 88]
  RT86.D45 2011
  610.73--dc22
                        2011008640
Second Printing, 2012

Publisher: Renee Wilmeth   **Principal Editor:** Carla Hall
Acquisitions Editor: Janet Boivin, RN   **Copy Editor:** Kate Shoup
Editorial Coordinator: Paula Jeffers   **Project Editor:** Billy Fields
Cover Designer: Studio Galou   **Proofreader:** Barbara Bennett
Interior Design and Page Composition: Rebecca Batchelor   **Indexer:** Jane Palmer

Dedication

This book is dedicated to all the colleagues I've had in the health care world since I first stepped through the doors of Lancaster General Hospital School of Nursing in 1971. The good ones have inspired, supported, humored, and kept me humble since my freshman class, when I was the last student to be passed on taking blood pressures. (God bless my instructor for taking me to have my hearing checked, rather than believing I just didn't realize that thumping sound was what I was supposed to be hearing.) The not-so-good associates have also taught me how to be better by showing me what I didn't want to be as a nurse.

Not coincidentally, my oldest and closest friends are those I met through the world of nursing, and if I didn't have them, I wouldn't be writing today. To my cousin, Shelba Purtle, who motivated me to become a nurse; to classmate Susan Kennel, who was dubbed along with me as "least likely to succeed;" to Sherry Lane, another graduate of LGH/1974; to Beth C., Kathleen, Kathy, Geri, Priscilla, Kendra, and many more I'll remember the instant this is cast in type—thank you for modeling the best that nursing has to offer.

Acknowledgements

I want to express special thanks to my children, Ellen and Joe Dellasega, who not only got ready for school without me on the many mornings when I had clinicals but also helped with typing and proofreading this manuscript when the time crunch hit. They both have the kind hearts of nurses, and I can imagine either or both of them being an excellent RN or CRNP one day. Also to little Blaire, my granddaughter, who gave up time with me so I could work on my book and who played the "Quiet Game" until Omee was done typing one more chapter. She, too, would make an excellent nurse in the future.

Although he is not alive to see this published, my late husband, Paul, celebrated every accomplishment and did all he could to support me in my writing and academic career. I still feel it, OAO, even if you're not right here.

About the Author

Cheryl Dellasega earned her PhD in health education and counseling and has worked clinically as a nurse practitioner. She is an expert on relational aggression (RA), a form of bullying used by females. She is the author of five nonfiction books on issues affecting women: *Forced to be Family* (Wiley, 2007), *Mean Girls Grown Up* (Wiley, 2005), *The Starving Family* (Champion Press, 2005), *Girl Wars* (Simon & Schuster, 2003), and *Surviving Ophelia* (Perseus, 2001). In 2007, Dellasega's young adult fiction series, *Bloggrls,* was launched by Marshall Cavendish. Dellasega's speaking, writing, and teaching offer essential insights into the different conflicts that arise within the context of female friendships and family relationships.

Table of Contents

Appendixes

Foreword

The idea that hospital nurses often aggressively bully each other probably shocks readers who are not in health care, but feels all too familiar to anyone who is. We nurses are acutely aware of the problem, but often have very little idea how the behavior gets set in motion, or what can be done to stop it. *When Nurses Hurt Nurses* helps with both situations—understanding where nurse bullying originates, and offering ideas for how to stop nurses from bullying each other.

Nurse bullying incidents are the result of "RA," or relational aggression; victims of such behavior can suffer from "PTED," or Post-Traumatic Embitterment Disorder. These acronyms may sound like jargon, but they serve an important purpose. Having technical-theoretical terms available to describe the kinds of on-the-job harassment nurses inflict on each other elevates those incidents to the level of a serious problem.

I have heard more than one nurse manager dismiss the meanness of nurses by saying, "That's just what happens when women work together." Using a term such as RA makes clear from the beginning that nurses being aggressively hostile at work is a serious problem that needs to be understood and effectively addressed by management.

The statistics quoted in the book put the incidence of nurse-on-nurse bullying between 40 and 70%. The reason people outside health care should feel concern about this figure is that bullying leads to poor communication, which ultimately compromises the ability of health care providers to work as teams. The end result is that patient care can become less safe.

"Safe" is almost a mantra we learn in nursing school. "Safe" is the bar below which no nurse may work. And yet, from my own experience working on a floor with a high degree of RA, I can say definitively that bullying among nurses creates an unsafe environment for nurses, and therefore patients. On my floor, asking a question would often be met with a sneer and a condescending, "You don't know *that*?" For obvious reasons, that response made me much less likely to ask questions. The nurses on the floor also ran in cliques, meaning that they tended to only help the nurses they considered friends. I remember times when I was drowning on the floor as a new nurse, and other nurses would not only *not* help, but would aggressively point out to me the many things I needed to finish.

Reading this, some people might say I had a rough work environment, but in the grand scheme of things, does it really matter? Yes, it does. It matters because it creates an unsafe environment for *patients*. A survey from *Critical Care Nurse* (2007) found nurses rated communication and collaboration as excellent 14% and 21% of the time, respectively. Dellasega explained why these figures matter: "Considering that these nurses worked in an environment where every aspect of nursing care could literally kill a patient, these results are abysmal. In any other industry, they would be unacceptable."

RA in hospitals can be dangerous for patients in the short term, and in the long term it negatively impacts the entire nursing profession. Every new nurse has a million and one questions, and a certain amount of self-doubt since the job has such an awesome level of responsibility. To keep nurses on the job, we need to create as nurturing an environment as possible to allow them to grow in competence and confidence. On a floor charged with RA, the opposite will happen: "One of the hardest things for victims is to understand that their tormenter's accusations have little to do with the truth. Indeed, this is why relational aggression is so powerful. Any nurse with the slightest crack in her self-esteem tends to personalize an aggressor's putdowns. If you are a new nurse [RA] can really hit hard."

One of the strengths of this book is that it looks at all parties involved in RA. Does the nurse manager play favorites and demoralize the staff by sending nasty e-mails? Do floor nurses pass on gossip unthinkingly, unaware of the personal damage they might cause? And most importantly, what is the role of the bystander?

Bystanders are the nurses who watch one nurse hassling another and either say nothing, or show solidarity with the bully by snickering. They are not directly dishing out harassment, but they also do not walk away, and thus they empower the abusive nurse by giving her a supportive audience. After reading this book, I decided to double my resolve never to be a bystander. I know I would never stand by silently while one nurse publicly berated another, but I also know I have listened to gossip and said nothing, instead of stressing that the nurses on the floor need to always support each other.

The ultimate strength of this book is that it shows how pervasive and endemic the problem of nurse-on-nurse bullying is. Reading it, and taking the few quizzes it contains, made me realize how inured I have become to aggression on the job. The really sad piece is that I have also stopped thinking about how RA could be addressed systemically. I try to always model the behavior I wish we all had, but I don't look for answers from above.

This book gave me some hope that change is possible, by showing that the first step is really to understand the problem. Dellasega invoked Maslow's well-known Hierarchy of Needs to explain that bullies have their own confidence issues and worries about job security. Nurses engaging in RA lash out from a sense of vulnerability, but sadly, they also have little interest in learning a different path: "A chronic master aggressor is struggling to protect her self-esteem and safety needs in every way she can think of. It's not likely she'll be reading a new book on being a better nurse in her off hours."

To paraphrase a famous quotation, "I have met the enemy, and she is us." RA thrives in hospitals because nurses feel powerless and overworked. The bully will not give thought to being a kinder nurse, but those of us who remain committed to the job can do that work ourselves, and then act accordingly. If we focus on helping each other, rather than hurting each other, it might make a world of difference.

—Theresa Brown, RN
Oncology nurse, author, and regular contributor
to the *New York Times* blog *Well*

Introduction

Recently, there has been much attention paid to the "mean girl" syndrome among adolescent girls. Gossip, exclusion, disloyalty, humiliation, manipulation, and intimidation are tools of the trade, and now, thanks to technology, young women can use relational aggression (female bullying) to hurt each other 24/7. Cyberbullying (text messages, blogs, polling booths, and other social media) offers yet another venue to anonymously strike out at other girls.

Among youth, relational aggression (RA) has negative outcomes that can last a lifetime; episodes of suicide have even been reported among young women who were targeted relentlessly by such behaviors. After writing a book about these behaviors (*Girl Wars*, Simon & Schuster, 2003), I was often asked: "What about adult women? Don't they use RA too?" and, "If a girl uses RA in middle school, will she keep on using it throughout her life?" In an effort to answer these questions, my next book, *Mean Girls Grown Up* (Wiley, 2005), collected narratives from a diverse group of adult women that suggested these behaviors continued in and out of the workplace, at the gym, in parent-school organizations, within community service groups, and even in places of worship (Dellasega, 2005).

As I gave talks and workshops on the book to various groups of women, the topic of nurses frequently surfaced. Over and over I heard, "They're the worst!" "You want to see some really bad behavior—study nurses!" "Go to a hospital for a day and you'll see the textbook on relational aggression!" Of course, as they say, I'd been there, done that, and gotten the T-shirt, but my story wasn't for public consumption just then.

In 2005, I began offering workshops and talks about RA specifically for nurses—often cathartic, usually painful, and hopefully helpful. During the course of these events, I began to hear story after story about the many ways in which nurses hurt each other using behaviors similar to the girls who attended my Club Ophelia programs (www.clubophelia.com). Dr. Diana Mason, at that time the editor of the *American Journal of Nursing* (*AJN*), encouraged me to write an article about what I knew.

That article, "Bullying Among Nurses," appeared in the January 2009 issue of *AJN*. In the weeks after it ran, I received 60 e-mails and many verbal comments from nurses who had read and agreed with the article. Not one e-mail of dispute or disagreement arrived. Here are just a few of the messages I got:

> *I manage two units and see this behavior frequently. I have had a speaker come in and talk about horizontal workplace violence, but to address it for what it is—"bullying"—I think makes a very strong point. In fact I have to discipline a nurse today for her bully behavior that caused disruption on the unit recently. I am a fairly new manager, and one unit in particular has been very aggressive, with a long history of bullying, and they have never had their poor behavior formally addressed before.*

* * *

> *Bravo! I have just reread your article. Thank you for covering this topic so beautifully. It's my perception*

that this horizontal violence among nurese is a long-standing yet unspoken sin. We also seem to underestimate the impact of this problem.

I just read your article, and I found it very interesting. There were different ways to bully that I didn't know about. Now I can identify those behaviors, and I find myself sometimes bullying others without knowing it. Thanks to your article, I will try to do better and to be careful to not hurt other people with whom I am working. There was a section written by Mrs. Durdock about "Bullying in the ICU" that expresses the feelings I had when I was working in the ICU unit. Reading your article does make me feel better, and better understand the things that are happening around me. Thank you very much. It means a lot to me.

* * *

I have witnessed this behavior in nursing at all levels of practice and in every specialty area. As a nursing instructor, I was so appalled by the behavior of students to each other that I implemented an activity for seniors in our new curriculum. It has been very therapeutic to many as they have verbalized how they have been personally affected. One thing that did not stop is how they treat each other, and I just wish I could do more to effect change among them. One of the graduating students is a victim of domestic violence and told me that she is essentially ostracized by her peers, save for one who gave her money and said, "You look like you need a hug." I felt so bad for her!

What's going on here? Caring or cruel? Are nurses just a self-selected bunch of women who somehow manage to switch their behavior on and off, going from kindness to meanness in a matter of moments? Or is something else to blame?

This book is meant to answer that question and to promote an understanding of RA, a form of social bullying, that creates so many problems it has almost become a hallmark of nursing—one of the professions the public trusts most. All names or potentially identifying details in vignettes or narratives have been changed to maintain confidentiality. Each chapter has an exercise at the end to build upon the information presented in the text—you might like to keep a journal as you read to jot down notes and write out the exercises.

I believe there are legitimate reasons why nurses take on the roles of aggressor, bystander, and victim. In addition, I know there are things we can do to turn behaviors around and make life better for everyone involved—which means better patient care, more attractive work environments, and, most importantly, higher quality of life for nurses.

–Cheryl Dellasega, PhD, CRNP

1 | RN RA: nurses and relational aggression

1 | women at work

In 2009, the U.S. Department of Labor reported that 59.2% of women over the age of 16 were either working or seeking work—a dramatic change from previous years, when women were expected to stay at home once they married. The largest percentage of these employed women (40%) worked in professional jobs. Secretarial and administrative positions were still the number one category, with nursing coming in second (U.S. DOL, 2009).

However, there was also a notable increase in female executives, and Berman (2010) reports that jobs considered "nontraditional" for women two decades ago are now held by a sizable percentage of females for instance, chemists, lawyers, and physicians. This introduces an element of competition for promotions—being judged by traditionally male standards, and still being among the minority gender. Consequently, one reason the type of relational aggression (RA) seen in corporate America differs from RA in the nursing field.

It is worth noting that 45 job categories remain where women make up less than 5% of employees. This means that for the many women working in non-nursing jobs, the opportunities for advancement, transfers, or executive opportunities are rare. Few role models or mentors exist. Therefore, the literature on corporate struggles among women is difficult to compare to scholarly work on nurses.

Heim, Murphy, and Golant (2010) found that women were more likely to undermine and bully each other in the workplace than to target a man. In the executive world, there are often conflicts over who gets promoted or has power and who doesn't, who is part of the power clique and who isn't, and who receives "favors" from the boss or supervisor and who doesn't. Even looks can play a role. There is also less male-male RA.

One executive commented that he sees women destroy each other in the workplace more often than he sees men mistreat women. In a series of articles in *Essence* magazine, African-American female executives discussed bullying they experienced at the hands of other African-American women as compared to discrimination and bullying from non–African-American women. Several on the panel felt that more problems occurred within the group than outside it.

Some Surprising Facts

Some information I collected as part of work with female professionals gave me the opportunity to dig a little deeper on the subject of RA and its impact. About 60 women shared their opinions. Part of their feedback is presented here:

- When asked how common they thought bullying was in the workplace between adult women, 73% answered "common" or "very common."

- In their opinion, 16% of the women they worked with were bullies, 27% were victims, and 39% were bystanders.

- They estimated that in the last week, they were a victim 1.8 times, a bully 1.5 times, and a bystander 6.8 times.

- When asked whether they had ever left a job because of bullying, 18% answered "yes."

- When asked whether they had ever missed a day of work because of bullying, 18% answered "yes."

- Some women had even experienced physical violence with another woman they worked with.

Aren't Nurses Just Like Everyone Else?

How does all this relate to RA and bullying within the nursing profession? There are several dynamics that lead nurses to label themselves differently than the female "bully bosses" found in non-nursing positions. Some are shaped by public opinion, but others come from within our own ranks.

The Worth of a Nurse

As the caring profession, nursing has long been one of the two acceptable "careers" for women (teaching being the other). The distinguished history of nursing and the many contributions made by nurses to improve global health were not reasons would-be RNs were guided into nursing school throughout the 20th century. Rather, it was because nursing would prepare them to be a good mother, provide a possible husband, and offer a reasonable income until a young woman got married.

Consider these excerpts from *A Collection of Nursing Stories* (1979), a book whose cover features a smiling blonde woman in a blue uniform. In the background are a stethoscope, a bottle of pills, and a handsome man cuddling a cat wrapped up in a blanket.

"So, you're a nurse?" said his wife, and led me to a corner, where she questioned me with a kind of detached pity, as if I had been an unmarried mother. After a struggle between disinclination and her duty as a social worker, she fixed a date for me to dine on my evening off....

—Monica Dickens

I think that the ideal nurse is one who understands what physical comfort will give her patient more peace of mind—little things like cooling the room, the furniture arranged so that it's restful to look at— when to talk and when not to—flowers on the tray, all that.

—Helen Dore Boylston, author of the
Sue Barton, Student Nurse *series*

But whatever happened, Hester was expected to have the breakfast things cleared away, and the ward ready for when the day nurses came on duty. Nurse Ridley's accusing eyes seemed to miss nothing, and Hester often wondered what it would be like to work under her unsympathetic supervision.

—Gordon Cooper

Even the full stories in the book that talk about male nurses portrayed them in an unexciting fashion, as this excerpt illustrates. The dialogue takes place between Jay, a female student nurse and a male classmate:

> *"Is it?" Jay asked. "Well, how come ever since Sister Clarke announced her retirement you've been going on about how it's the ideal job for a male nurse?"*
>
> *"Because it is."*
>
> *"Meaning a woman can't do it just as well?"*
>
> *"You said it."*

Are We "Don't Want to Bees"?

With these stereotypes, it's hard to feel proud about the nursing profession. As pointed out by Gordon (2010) the lack of "voice" that nurses are prone to and their feelings that being paid for caring about and for sick people somehow reveals a lack of integrity. (In contrast, curing, the physician's purview, is a perfectly legitimate way to make a living.)

The public image of nurses hasn't done much to enhance professional self-esteem, either. Kalisch and Kalisch (1986) describe television commercials and movies that portray nurses as either sexy sluts or hard-hearted bullies (think Nurse Ratched in *One Flew Over the Cuckoo's Nest* by Ken Kesey, starring

Jack Nicholson). When you are part of a group that has traditionally come in second best to physicians and has all the other aforementioned baggage, it's no surprise many bypass it as a career, despite their interest—although many also return to it in later years. There is already a sense of being underappreciated and perhaps a bit mistreated by the public at large. Has the traditional lack of power nurses experience in the health care system made us reluctant to pursue a leadership role? Have we become "Don't want to bees"? or, worse yet, "Afraid to bees"?

Add to that working circumstances in which you may not eat, sit down, or go to the bathroom for long periods, and the stressors mount. Then there's the fact that unlike other workplaces, most nurses can't leave and take a break when emotions run high or the atmosphere on the unit is tense. Not only must you stay and keep working, you must focus on patients who depend on you to make them feel better, not vice versa.

I've never met a nurse who doesn't express her frustrations. Lucy, a 30-year-old RN with 10 years of experience, noted "Nurses work in a pressure-cooker environment. You walk in the door of the hospital and it slams behind you, and off you go to navigate the maze of your day, which is too intense 95 percent of the time." Will nursing ever be stereotyped as a glamorous career? Are nurses ever going to feel blessed instead of bitter about the job they chose?

It's not surprising to hear nurses complain, but it's taken too long for a dialogue to begin about what happens when tensions and pressures reach overload. The stakes are higher for our profession than in many others, yet until recently, nurses have accepted the "eating your young" phenomenon as if it's just another part of the licensing exam.

As a profession, an organization, or an individual, we have the power to change the emotional environment we work in every day. If you're happy to trudge along using the same behaviors and getting the same results, you'll probably be able to manage just that. But if you picked this book up hoping it would help you improve your quality of work life, read on, knowing that tomorrow can be different.

Exercise

Talk to another nurse about the public image of nursing. Is it becoming more positive with newer, more realistic television shows about nursing and nurses in positions of power? Or are we still portrayed negatively? Do nurses in these shows use relational aggression against each other, or are they more likely to be bullied by physicians?

2 | the caring profession

Nursing was not my first choice of a career, but I grew to love it with each new stage of development: going from diploma nurse, to BSN, then on to obtaining graduate and nurse practitioner degrees, and finally my PhD. Those were only rungs on the educational ladder, though. Along with all the classroom schooling on nursing, the most valuable lessons I learned were about suffering people and the nursing culture. Never was I taught how to listen or communicate effectively, and I certainly never heard bullying discussed.

As a new nurse, I saw a coworker treat a patient incredibly kindly and then walk out of the patient's room and rip a colleague to shreds with her words. In the ICU, nurses jockeyed for recognition as the smartest and most accomplished "supernurse." When I returned to school, there was a different kind of competition: to see who could excel at nursing both in and out of the classroom.

When I worked on my doctorate and taught under-graduate students, an invisible but impermeable barrier separated the master's degree faculty clique from the PhD clique. There was also a division between hospital workers ("real nurses") and teachers ("up in their ivory towers").

Once I earned my PhD, nurses in clinical settings regarded me as unrealistic and unprepared for real nursing—until they discovered I worked one day a week as a nurse practitioner. Tenure-track expectations were just another form of competition and another chance for my colleagues to pore over a candidate's dossier and find fault with their performance. It seemed there was no end to the different relationally aggressive behaviors displayed by nurses, but no one seemed to consider it unusual or problematic. By then (the 1980s), courses and workshops on therapeutic touch and assertive communication had begun to emerge, but no one looked at nurses and thought we needed help with our relationships with each other.

The RA That Drove Me Away

Then came the act of aggression that led me to leave my position in nursing and go to a completely different college. During my years on tenure-track, I naturally did a lot of writing. True, it wasn't the creative fiction I had dreamed of writing during my high-school years. Even so, it was something I was good at, and soon my publication list was impressive.

What I was proudest of was my collaboration record. After completing the required number of first and solo-authored articles in scholarly journals, I was quick to make sure my graduate students and colleagues got published too. I'll never forget a bulletin board put up one year to track faculty publications. The majority of them were mine, and at least 85% were with other nursing faculty in the same school.

When my chairperson arranged for an appointment with me that spring, I felt sure she was going to compliment me for helping others in the school. (My efforts went beyond co-authorships and included grants and other projects.) Imagine my shock when she smiled and told me she felt I just wasn't a "team player." She went on to say that she had "heard rumors" I was "critical of nursing to other departments across campus." When I asked who had told her such rumors, she quietly declined to reveal her sources. Later, I would learn this is a typical RA tactic: refusing to reveal sources of information because there really aren't any.

Things hadn't been enjoyable for me professionally for some time, but in the aftermath of her confrontation—which I discovered was only RA attack one (undermining and misrepresenting)—it turned out her confrontation had been partially orchestrated by another faculty member who thought I had my eye on her job (RA attack two: gossip and misrepresenting comments she had elicited). Like many of the abused women I had worked with in clinical situations, I finally asked myself why I was staying in a situation that chipped away at my self-esteem day after day. It was time for a sabbatical from the situation. It hurt to think I had "failed" at something so important to me, but the double sabotage was the *coup de grâce* in a hostile environment that had already led to several resignations and would lead to several more after mine. (Ironically, everyone who left went on to happier and more successful positions.)

PTED: Not Just Me

At a recent conference, one speaker described a condition that most of us were not familiar with: Post-Traumatic Embitterment Disorder (PTED). Dr. Michael Linden (2003) authored a paper about the disorder, which is similar to Post-Traumatic Stress Disorder (PTSD). Patients with PTSD display symptoms after a pivotal near-death event, becoming anxious and fearful. Similarly, people with PTED function normally and are healthy mentally and physically until a distressing event shatters their lives, causing them to question all that they had believed in and valued to that point.

As I write about the RA environment that led to a turning point in my professional life, I believe I and many of my colleagues suffered from PTED. We had been educated to believe that if we worked hard and obtained the right graduate degrees, our efforts would be valued. Instead, a particularly toxic coworker working in tandem with an undermining boss placed us in a pressure cooker of constant uncertainty and fearfulness.

Surprisingly, a new opportunity presented itself more quickly than I might have anticipated. It was one that allowed me some time off before starting, so I was able to do some of the creative writing I enjoyed, as well as author the book *Surviving Ophelia* (2001), which was my first commercial endeavor. That book wasn't about bullying and relational aggression directly, but it did help me further understand the importance of female relationships and the hurt that accumulates when things go wrong between mothers and daughters.

Book by book, experience by experience, I've come to the point of understanding many of the dynamics involved in relational aggression. That doesn't mean I accept it, sanction it, or believe it is inevitable. Quite the opposite: I've started programs for young girls (http://www.clubophelia.com) that help me believe these behaviors can and must change. In my work with nurses on this topic, I'm often told that this is impossible, that "nothing will ever change." Again, I don't believe that's true.

Nurses are in the caring profession. There are theories about nursing as a career; remember the nursing-theory lectures of Jean Watson and Madeleine Leininger, who both found the concept so vital they structured their beliefs around it (Vance, 2003)? Taber (1993) lists the top 10 caring behaviors nurses display as "attentive listening, comforting, honesty, patience, dependability, providing information, touch, sensitivity, respect, and honoring the patient." Leininger (1991) believes that caring is not only the focus of nursing, it is what unifies the nursing profession. We learn this as students, but we don't learn what to do when those around us act in distinctly uncaring ways. Leadership content in most nursing curricula covers a range of topics relevant to management and professionalism, but despite encouragement from our accrediting bodies to have zero tolerance for RA, no one spells out how this looks in real life.

It's Not All Bad!

Recently, at a lecture I gave, one woman in the audience timidly raised her hand and asked if there was anything good going on in nursing. It was disappointing, because I thought I had emphasized that although RA is a problem, no one will support or help you like another nurse. When I challenge nurses in my workshops to list random and not-so-random acts of kindness they've seen from other nurses, the lists are mind-boggling. They cite nurses who give up their day off to another nurse who is ill; nurses who donate time, money, and emotional support when a crisis occurs; nurses who compliment and celebrate accomplishments; and much more. It seems that for every story I've heard of extreme negative behavior, there's at least one that involves an equal degree of goodness.

I believe things don't have to be the way they were for me or how other nurses described them. If a change is to occur, however, it needs to start during the formative years of a nurse's education. We need to continue with workshops and seminars on healthy and respectful relationship skills. Instead of tearing each other down, we need to build each other up.

Maybe I'm just an optimist, though. After a recent eight-hour workshop with nurses, one attendee remained behind. When we were alone, she came forward and leaned on the speaker's podium. "That was a great program," she said. "But I've been a nurse for 20 years, and it's always 'Do this,' and 'Do that.' Nothing ever changes." She continued, with a look of disbelief on her face, "Nurses are mean. That's just the way it is. Nothing's going to change."

As she chugged off, the conference conveners, who had been collapsing chairs and gathering up evaluations behind her, looked at me and rolled their eyes. I couldn't help watching the woman make her way out the door.

What would it be like to work with someone who refused to believe change was even possible?

http://www.ourownworstenemies. com

Yet, the same kinds of negative stories about nurse aggression abound on the Internet. The website allnurses. com (http://allnurses.com) includes a forum on "The Bully Nurse," with 10 posts about "What makes a bully nurse?" A summary of the responses sound like a textbook description of relational aggression: She (always female) is: overly critical, arrogant, bossy, jealous, competitive, evaluates others negatively, puts others on the spot constantly, creates cliques, and takes pleasure in humiliating colleagues. Check out the website AboutMyTalk.com (http://www. aboutmytalk.com) and you'll find that 85% of respondents agreed that "Nurses thrive on backstabbing each other." In the posts that follow the poll, examples of such behavior are shared.

"What Really Gets Me About Nursing"

Then there's IHateNursing.com (http://www.ihatenursing.com), a forum for dissatisfied nurses to support fellow nurses, effect change, and inform the world what being a nurse really is all about. The site is a free-for-all for complaints about being around other nurses. These quotes say it all:

I can withstand the nasty docs, the nasty pts, the odors, the paperwork, the drudgery, the 12 hrs with no food, etc. But what I can't stand is walking into the nurses' station and just being either glared at or ignored by a bunch of TOADS who must hate their jobs so much they can't even muster a decent conversation. I mean, these are SUPPOSED to be my colleagues—my peers!

***

The managers, promoted by relation/friendship, not merit, do not back up their own nurses. Quite the opposite. Steady flows of "nasty grams" let you know you didn't refill the ice pitcher in room 450 on the day you were understaffed by 17 hours.

***

I'm absolutely dried up, washed out, and burnt to a crisp. I got into the game when I was 17 as an assistant while I worked my way through university. I don't know WHAT I thought I was working toward. I'm 25 now, and realize that I have an absolute joke for a "profession" and have to spend all my working life with vile, malevolent, evil, and malicious bitches. I'm in law school now, but it's a shame that my career to this point has been wasted.

This narrative, from my book *Mean Girls Grown Up* (Wiley, 2005), illustrates the specific types of relational aggression one nurse experienced:

> *Oh my! The nursing profession! I have been in it for seventeen years. I was nineteen when I started working in a local hospital where I was loved and nurtured. God blessed me with that job. After two years, I took a position with another local hospital ... There wasn't much nurturing there, but I have always felt that the nursing profession does eat its young! Over the years there continues to be backstabbing, gossiping, rumor starting, eye rolling, whispering, and exclusion.... We even have a nursing supervisor who exhibits relational aggression all the time. It is not uncommon for someone to say, "She is stirring the trouble pot again." (p. 91)*

Is Anyone Giving Compliments?

That doesn't mean that there aren't websites or blogs out there that extol the benefits of nursing. Elizabeth Songer (http://www.associatedcontent.com/article/399286/ top_ten_reasons) wrote "Top Ten Reasons I Love Being a Registered Nurse," but added "Plus Five Reasons It Kinda Sucks." Lippincott's NursingCenter.com (http:// www.nursingcenter.com) managed to garner three positive comments about nursing when they put out a call asking, "Do you love nursing?"

However, in a classic case of online RA, an LPN who wrote about her love for nursing on the site AboutMyJob.com (http://www.aboutmyjob.com) was roundly slammed by commenters who chided her for considering herself a nurse when RNs are the "real nurses." Ironically, the commenters went on to claim, "80% of the problem with nursing is what WE do to each other."

So even when nurses try to be positive and upbeat about their career choice, it seems their colleagues knock them down. What is it that happens between the time when a student nurse steps into his or her first class and the point where comments like these are posted on the Internet for all to see?

Educated to Aggress?

As I write this, two members of my family are in training to be nurses. Both are sweet and good-hearted, with hope for the future and a willingness to help others in any way possible. Like most of their peers, they are going into nursing because they care about people. Ask their classmates what attracted them to the profession, and I suspect almost all will say the same thing: "I want to help people," or "I'm a caring person." Most medical students have the same motivation for entering medicine. Yet somehow, between that first day of class and the day of graduation, I see students change. Yes, they are still caring—but not to each other, as demonstrated in these examples:

- Students obtaining study notes from classes the year before and using them as bargaining chips for friendships

- Certain students who were outcasts because they didn't fit the mold of the majority in terms of clothing, hairstyle, and disposable income being ridiculed by their classmates

- Students who acted nice to a classmate's face but nasty behind her back

- Students who harassed and threatened certain instructors over grades—not because they cared about their grade, but to give teachers they didn't like a hard time

Students used other subtle behaviors to put each other down, such as spreading rumors, gossiping, and engaging in online aggression. But these paled in comparison to what happened at certain hospitals where they gained their clinical experience. Suddenly, the roles they played were reversed. The students were on the receiving end of mean behavior. Experienced nurses would hide laundry, snarl at students, refuse to answer their questions, make fun of them to coworkers, and question the value of a "fancy college degree." If any of the instructors tried to intervene, the hospital nurses would stand with their arms folded and their eyes rolled, acting as if students who complained about their behavior just weren't tough enough to be "real nurses." Then there were the instructors who felt the best way to teach was to intimidate. Foster et al. (2004) found that 90% of students reported being bullied by their instructors, while Edwards and O'Connell (2006) noted that nurse educators often use bullying techniques to teach because they mistakenly believe fear will motivate learning.

It would be a relief to think these types of negative behaviors are part of the educational process and end once the school years are over. Unfortunately, that's not the case. Nurses across the country have shared their stories of relational aggression with me, and claim that RA is the reason so many in our profession burn out early.

In the book *My First Year as a Nurse*, Naomi Shuster writes:

> *What I discovered is that your "fellow" nurses can really stick it to you in the back. Part of the problem lies in the hospital hierarchy. There are baccalaureate-trained nurses and LPNs. There are also nurses with master's degrees. Each group seems to resent the others. As for the doctors, they can scream at you for nothing. Everything bad is the nurse's fault. I think a hysterical*

doctor forces a nurse to cover her own behind, and she is often ready to blame another nurse just to protect herself. (p. 69)

Exercise

What experiences did you have as a student that were examples of relational aggression? Did you and your classmates ever learn about relational aggression in your courses? Give some examples of early experiences where other nurses helped or hindered your adjustment to nursing through their behavior and attitude.

3 | nurse against nurse? no way!

Teasing out the difference between nurse-to-nurse relational aggression and general bullying from all coworkers, including physicians, is a limitation of the existing studies on nurse bullying, most of which are European. Vessey (2007) says 44% of nurses report having experienced "peer bullying" at work within the last year, while Quine (2001) found a similar prevalence among nurses, which was 10% higher than in other work groups. Again, the source of the bullying is not specifically identified as nurse-to-nurse in either study.

Another report on 5,655 hospital employees by Kivimaki, Elovainio, and Vahtera (2000) showed 50% of nurses complained of being bullied at work, as compared to 8% of physicians. Alspach (2007) reports that among critical-care nurses, 18% of RNs had experienced verbal abuse from another RN, and 25 to 32% of RNs described their interactions with peers as fair or poor in quality.

Vessey et al. (2009) did find that when the right questions about bullying were asked, interesting differences about place and person emerged. From a convenience sample of 303 nurses, she discovered that 70% reported bullying had occurred to them. The most frequent sites were medical surgical units (23%), critical care (18%), emergency departments (12%), operating room/post-anesthesia care units (9%), and obstetrical units (7%). Aggressors were most often senior nurses (24%), charge nurses (17%), nurse managers (14%), and physicians (8%).

RNs and RA

Traditionally, the stereotype has been nurses being bullied involved a gruff, paternalistic physician who verbally demeaned nurses simply because he could. (And the physician was always a "he" in this historical version of aggression.) Stringer (2001) reports that 90% of nurses have been verbally abused, most often by physicians and frequently after a stressful incident. While the underlying reasons for abuse is not clear, hospitals do themselves a disservice by ignoring the issue, since 35% of nurses leave their jobs because of verbal abuse and 70% have said that abuse from physicians caused errors and reduced productivity. A report from the Health Policy and Economic Research Unit suggests that medical students identified doctors as the leading source of intimidation (23%). Surprisingly, however, nurses were their second most frequent nemesis (16.4%), meaning nurses are not always innocent victims—nor is there any reason to believe their bullying and RA has less onerous outcomes than that of physicians.

Vessey et al. (2001) said that when bullying occurs within a profession, it is "horizontal violence." Two recent studies from the U.S. suggest that nurses are likely to engage in "lateral" or "horizontal" violence. A 2006 survey of 4,000 critical-care nurses found that 18% had been verbally abused by another nurse, and more than 25% rated the quality of their communication and teamwork with other nurses as fair or poor (Ulrich, 2001). A study of new nurses at a Boston hospital found that half had lateral violence directed at them (Griffin, 2004).

Nurse Theresa Brown attracted attention when her essay, "When the Nurse Is a Bully," was published in the *New York Times*. After witnessing two incidents of nurses being mistreated by coworkers, she recalls a time when she was treated as if she "had a huge bull's-eye on my back," and says once that happened, it was hard to focus on her nursing work. She believes nurses turn on each other because they can't fight back and don't like to talk about problems openly. In the comments that follow Ms. Brown's article, an uncomfortable number are from patients who report being bullied by nurses.

In the literature, there is a general agreement that the term "horizontal" offers conceptual clarity because it seems to imply that nurses aggress against those in the same oppressed group as themselves. Kirkhorn et al. (2010) say, "The concept of workplace or horizontal violence is difficult to define as there are many terms that have been used interchangeably in the literature, such as: bullying, marginalization, verbal abuse, mobbing, and victimization" (p. 210). For these methodological reasons, determining how many nurses are actually mistreated by other nurses through RA or bullying is difficult because most surveys fail to ask who the aggressor is or specify what behaviors are being assessed. For example, is refusing to help a coworker get a patient out of bed because you don't like him or her the same as giving that person a verbal dressing down when there's a large crowd of spectators within hearing range?

Before a workshop I conducted on nurses and relational aggression, I collected some evaluation data by issuing a pretest for all enrolled participants. There were 46 female nurses and six males. They ranged in age from 23 to 65, with the average being 46. The average number of years of nursing experience was 19, but the range was from 3 to 45. Just seeing those last two demographics gives you an idea of how very different the nursing profession has become in terms of age, gender, and years of experience.

Now the RA data they provided:

- Relational aggression occurs most often in the healthcare profession as:
  - Physicians bullying nurses: 7%
  - Nurses bullying nurses: 82%
  - Physicians bullying physicians: 7%
  - Other: 10%
- Male doctors are more likely to use relational aggression against a female nurse than a female doctor.
  - Agree: 57%
  - Disagree: 43%
- Female doctors are more likely to use relational aggression against a female nurse than a female doctor.
  - Agree: 83%
  - Disagree: 16.7%
- Female nurses are more prone to relational aggression than male nurses.
  - Agree: 85%
  - Disagree: 13%
- I would describe myself as:
  - Aggressor: 2%

- Bystander: 13%

- Victim: 2%

- All: 42%

- None: 41%

From the answers to these questions, you can see that nurses felt RA is a female phenomenon, more likely to happen between women, and the most common form of aggression in healthcare.

For the Record...

How is relational aggression different from horizontal violence or bullying? RA is much more complex than abuse from one person or set of peers. Verbal and behavioral abuse can occur from coworkers of equal, lesser, or higher status; physicians, medical students, or residents; nurse supervisors or administrators; and so on. That means instead of slugging someone with your fist, you come up with a sharply worded zinger that will leave them humiliated and in tears. Or you may turn to a coworker and whisper something each time your target walks by and then laugh loud enough for her to hear.

It is a form of social bullying that's not much different from the kind of mean-girl behavior that goes on in middle school and high school, except now it's between grown women. (The consensus on men has yet to come in.)

Believe it or not, I have heard of this kind of aggression even turning physical, which of course resulted in major sanctions for both parties involved.

RA is often covert or subtle, so it can often be overlooked, disclaimed, or ignored by superiors who are in a position to help. It is often called by other names that have come to stereotype women in general:

- Female bullying
- Covert aggression
- Bitchy
- Catty
- Catfighting
- Drama

How Does RA Differ from Bullying?

What does RA behavior look like? When I run a workshop or give a lecture, I generally ask women to tell me about the RA behaviors they experience. Inevitably, the list looks something like this:

- Gossip
- Manipulation (getting someone to buy you things or do favors in a misleading way)

- Intimidation and threats ("If you don't stay away from my man, I'll...")

- Exclusion (intentionally leaving someone out of an event or conversation)

- Gestures/body language (rolling eyes, sighing, fake smiles)

- Ridicule or mean criticism meant to hurt

- Saying something mean and then pretending you were "joking"

- Name-calling

- Teasing/harassment, mean jokes about sensitive issues

- Cliques (similar to exclusion)

- Campaigns (turning one or more people against another)

- Shifting loyalties (being friends one day and enemies the next)

- Betraying confidences and giving away secrets

Don't forget the cyber-forms of RA. In addition to websites that spew general anger, there are other forms of online RA, such as the following:

- Polling booths (i.e., "Who is the dumbest employee?")

- Video clips that ridicule another
- Sharing of e-mails meant to be private
- Blogs where negative things about specific people are posted
- Facebook and other social media used to humiliate someone
- Nasty text messages, tweets, etc.
- Flame wars (ganging up on another nurse online)

If anything, online RA is often more vicious than real-time RA because the aggressor doesn't see her target's face when she delivers her hurtful message worldwide. Girls and women admit they feel less accountable for their words and behavior when there's a computer screen or cell phone between them and the person with whom they're communicating. For women, tone of voice, facial expression, head position, and eyebrow position are all embellishments to the message. They can turn a speaker's words from kind to cruel in an instant.

While it might seem as if RA is something most women have lived with since childhood, in reality, serious consequences can result from episodes that occurred long ago but which left what some women call "the deepest hurt." If the RA is part of everyday life, the outcomes can be even more severe. The following have been linked to job stress, if not specifically to RA (Almost & Laschinger, 2002; Boone, et al., 2008; Parsons & Stonestreet, 2004; Rosenstein & O'Daniel, 2005; Gauci-Borda & Norman, 2001; Kenkel, 2003; Manderino and Berkey, 1997; Parsons & Stonestreet, 2004):

- Burnout, frequent job turnovers, quitting before completing orientation

- Psychosomatic symptoms such as headaches, upset stomachs, frequent illness, and general malaise

- Depression and anxiety

- Low job satisfaction and powerlessness

- Other negative consequences: poor quality of life, reduced productivity, impaired relationships with coworkers

Certainly, RA is a form of bullying, which is why many refer to it as covert bullying or social bullying. But while bullying is often meant for public display and usually involves a power differentiation, RA can occur unobtrusively between any two women.

Nursing RA Behaviors

Over the years, my work with nurses has led me to believe they have their own unique ways of expressing RA that parallel the list of behaviors I shared earlier. Here are some of the ways nurses tell me aggression plays out in their work life:

- Giving another nurse "the silent treatment"

- Spreading rumors throughout the unit, hospital, or organization

- Humiliating or putting down another nurse, usually with regard to his or her nursing skills or abilities

- Failing to support another nurse because you don't like him or her (this could be anything from failing to help with care to disagreeing with decisions the nurse made)

- Failing to come to another nurse's assistance because you don't like him or her (a particular problem in emergency departments [EDs] and psychiatric units)

- Refusing to share information with another nurse or otherwise setting him or her up for failure

- Excluding another nurse from on- or off-the-job socializing

- Repeating information shared by one nurse out of context so it reflects badly on him or her

- Running a smear campaign or otherwise trying to get others to turn against another nurse

- Sharing a confidence you were asked to keep private and perhaps twisting it a bit out of context

- Making fun of another nurse's appearance, demeanor, or other trait

- Manipulating or intimidating another nurse into doing something for you

- Using body language (such as eye-rolling or head-tossing) to convey an unfavorable opinion of someone

- Saying something unfavorable, then pretending you were joking

- Name-calling

- Making a nurse look bad in front of patients, other nurses, or supervisors

- Teasing another nurse for his or her lack of skill or knowledge

In general, stress levels tend to rise during times of transition—even seemingly minor ones. Darla recalls this well. See how many of the aforementioned behaviors you can find in her story:

My patient, a 41-year-old IV drug user admitted for pneumonia, sat at the end of her bed screaming profanity, minutes after extubation, and using inappropriate hand gestures directed at me, her primary nurse. The pulmonologist felt this patient would be successful off the ventilator and wrote parameters to wean her oxygen using her pulse oximeter. When the male physician was at the bedside, the patient was calm, cooperative, and pleasant.

After he was out of sight, the screaming of profanity began—at me, her female nurse. There was a constant pulling at her IV sites and disconnecting heart monitor leads. The noise was disruptive to the unit, but my role was to unconditionally care for this disturbing patient and juggle my responsibility of also caring for my other patient—an elderly man with an inferior wall MI. I was thinking to myself, why did I ever want to be a nurse?

I noted my patient's voice was becoming hoarse and monitored her for respiratory distress. Leaving her door open, I walked to our supply area where I found a non-rebreather oxygen mask. Walking back to my patient's room, I saw the door to my patient's room was closed. The unit secretary reported that she saw our nurse manager close the door. She alone had been brave enough to confront her, saying, "I know the patient is disturbing, but please leave the door open so Darla can watch her, as she is not safe to be left alone." Since she was "just" a secretary, the nurse manager rolled her eyes and left the unit.

Amazingly, none of my nurse coworkers dared confront the manager, who was known for her temper. As the nurse, I knew my patient was scared and her screaming profanity was her way of crying out for help. Needless to say, the closed door increased her fear and made my job more difficult. I was too busy caring for my patient's needs to talk to my manager at the time. At the end of my shift, I went to her office and found a note that said, "Gone for the day."

I signed my nurse's notes that day with my name, RN, BSN. I was the nurse legally responsible for this critical care patient. The support and respect I received from my nurse manager was a closed door. She closed the door to the patient's disturbing profanity as well as to an opportunity to support a nurse in the unit she managed. Only the unit secretary had backed me up, and she wasn't even trained to understand what was needed most in the situation.

The next story is more subtle, because the RA dealt out came with a mix of what seemed to be kindness. Amy was a new graduate, working the night shift in the ICU. A few hours before the end of her shift, a nurse in charge of staffing informed her she was mandated to work four extra hours that morning because there weren't enough nurses to care for the patients. Although Amy had plans for lunch with her husband, she was told the charge nurse wasn't making a request; she was giving a directive. The extra hours left Amy exhausted. She worked 16 hours and returned for her next scheduled 12-hour shift on just a few hours of sleep.

At the end of her shift, Amy was greeted by her former preceptor, Jill. Jill gave Amy a warm, supportive hug and said, "Thank you, thank you, thank you!" Amy had no idea what Jill was talking about and asked her to explain. Jill told Amy that she was originally scheduled to work overtime the morning before, but when she called to ICU to see if she was needed, the charge nurse told her no, because Amy had graciously offered to work extra. Coincidentally, Jill and the charge nurse were close friends. Amy concludes her story by saying, "As a new graduate, this was my welcome to the caring profession of nursing."

When Does RA Occur?

There are certain times, such as holidays and summer vacations, when many workplaces experience a surge in RA behaviors. In hospitals or health care organizations, these can be exaggerated by the increase in illnesses that often accompany other seasonal issues and act as a catalyst for increased tension. Mergers, local plant closings that lead to unemployment for families of nurses, and a host of situational problems can add to the pressure-cooker environment most hospitals already function in. For other primary or chronic care facilities, the shockwaves aren't much different because there are fewer staff to absorb the impact of factors outside the health care organization that cause more tension for the nurses who work there.

I've been consulted by many hospitals in the wake of a major stressor. The situation usually looks something like this: A particular unit is short-staffed because of illness, reorganizing, a wave of layoffs or transfers, or any of a number of other reasons. As a result, nurses feel like they're working in a pressure cooker. New nurses are recruited and brought in, but the existing staff is so stressed, they are less than welcoming. In fact, some, if not many, of the nursing RA behaviors (described previously) are exhibited. Consequently, the new nurses exit as if they were in a revolving door.

Even holidays and vacations can provoke upset and stress. Units are usually working with reduced numbers of personnel to accommodate vacations. On top of that, everyone is engaged in extra activities, such as shopping for gifts, travel planning, and arranging get-togethers to attend after work. This mix of excitement, fatigue, and anxiety can cause tempers to flare and behavior meltdowns to increase. Other situations like romantic interests on the unit, illness, family stressors, new administrators, or new policies can also have a negative impact.

Stringer (2001) reports that workplace abuse increases nursing turnover and exacerbates the shortage of nurses. Interestingly, two-thirds of nurses in her report said abuse escalates after a stressful incident. Another study showed a 50% higher rate of absence from work among those who had been bullied (Kivimaki, Elovainio, & Vahtera, 2000).

Underneath It All

There are approximately 3.1 million registered nurses in the United States, with only 5.4 to 5.7% of these nurses being male (HRSA, 2010, CAN, 2008). Some experts believe that because nursing is a female-dominated profession, it is not surprising to find RA behaviors creating a toxic work environment.

Women are relationship-oriented. We crave relationships as children and are broken-hearted if we don't have the right ones as teens and often as adults. While men usually consider their wives to be their best friend, women turn to their female pals for this role. For many reasons, nurses count on each other for help. Yet all too often, competition and mistrust prevent them from truly collaborating with each other (Hutchinson, Vickers, Jackson, & Wilkes, 2005).

In a follow-up to a previous survey, the editors of *Critical Care Nurse* (2007) found that 14% of nurses rated the quality of communication between RNs on their work units as excellent, 17% rated the collaboration as excellent, and 21% rated respect for others as excellent. Considering that these nurses worked in an environment where every aspect of nursing care could literally kill a patient, these results are abysmal. In any other industry they would be unacceptable. Can you imagine flying in a plane in which the flight attendants feel that only 14% of their communication is excellent? One has to hope that action was taken to improve communication, collaboration, and respect among the nurses, (as well as the other health care team members) after this study.

If nurses on a unit or work team aren't communicating well with each other, they're much more likely to communicate poorly with patients, supervisors, and physicians—a chief cause of errors in hospitals. Feeling unsafe and having low professional self-esteem are also negative outcomes of RA that can spill over to affect a nurse's personal life.

Exercise

Look at the list of nursing RA behaviors in this chapter and count how many of them you used on your last full shift at work. Try to figure out if you are prone to putting other nurses down without even realizing it through a particular behavior. If so, see if you can figure out what triggers this behavior. Is it fatigue, frustration, or perhaps a particular coworker?

Take a second look at the list and see if others have used these behaviors against you. If so, how did you feel when it happened? Can you pinpoint what led up to the meltdown? What might you do differently if the situation were to occur again?

4 | bosses aren't the only bullies

Childers (2004) shares several stories of nursing situations that involve "freak physicians and out-of-control supervisors," but suggests that other factors play a role in the bullying dynamic. All too often, the overly aggressive "queen bee," her target(s), and the "bystander bees" aren't quite as obvious as Childers would have us believe.

The Bully

The aggressor or bully can be one or more nurses. While any one of us on any given day can act more aggressively than we would like, to be truly caught in the rut of RA, a bully nurse will *constantly* use aggressive behaviors. It won't matter whether she is at lunch, walking to her car, or working in her office; she is in attack mode. She conveys her outlook through body language as well as words. Every nurse on the floor knows the meaning of her raised eyebrows and heavy sigh. If there's a group of aggressors, the venom increases exponentially until the entire environment turns toxic.

Take Janet, my second nurse manager back in the era when specialty units were new creatures. Most everyone who worked on our unit was a little intimidated by the heart monitors and IV-regulating equipment. Although Janet could have been the ideal educator—she was older than most of us, and more experienced overall—that's not what happened.

Janet "adopted" me as her pet. She quickly told me how terrible all the other nurses were. She wasted no time pointing out their mistakes and humiliating them in front of other nurses (usually me, her constant, albeit unwilling, companion). "Look at this," she would sneer, loudly paging the nurse involved over the patient call system. When the culprit arrived, Janet would point out all the mistakes the nurse had made: knotted monitor leads, tangled IV tubing, and strips of EKG monitor paper that the doctors had left behind on the bed table. I would look away, embarrassed to be a witness to the other nurse's humiliation but helpless to intervene. Still in my orientation period, I was even more vulnerable to Janet's potential bullying, so I kept silent as she trashed one nurse after the other.

Eventually, Janet and I parted ways. All it took was one incident in which I stood up to her and said, "No." She quickly dropped me as her protégé. I've long since forgotten the particulars, but I do remember that Janet was acting like her typical self, and I finally got tired of it. Once I told her that her criticism of another nurse was wrong and gave her proof that I was correct, it was as if we had never met. She treated me like a total stranger from that day on.

Eventually, our nurse supervisor caught on to Janet's management style and moved her to the night shift, where she discovered a group of nurses who had worked together for a long time. They weren't about to let Janet ruin their collegiality. When she couldn't drop her bullying style in order to fit in, she quickly found herself a loner.

I felt sorry for Janet. One day, I ran across her walking toward her car in the parking lot. I stopped and expressed regret for the way things had turned out between us. I had learned a lot from her, I said, and appreciated her years of experience. Janet looked at me with blank eyes and said nothing. Then she turned and walked in the other direction, cutting off the rest of the conversation. Would I have had the courage to tell her that she came across a little too strong, and that's why virtually every nurse treated her like a pariah? I don't know.

The Victim

Usually, the bully's target, or victim, has done nothing to invoke the aggression being directed her way—at least not intentionally. Unfortunately, most nurses who are treated as someone else's personal bull's-eye feel exactly the opposite, which is not unusual. After all, they are the ones who just got hammered verbally or ridiculed with a roll of the eyes.

One of the hardest things for victims is to understand that their tormentors' accusations have little to do with the truth. Indeed, this is why relational aggression is so powerful. Any nurse with the slightest crack in her self-esteem tends to personalize an aggressor's put-downs. If you are a new nurse, a nurse who has just transferred to a different unit, a nurse experiencing troubles at home, and so on, being criticized in front of a group of nurses for your work, your personal appearance, your educational background, or any of a number of other things by a bully coworker can really hit hard.

Susan is a good example. Susan always stayed at work until the tasks for her evening shift were complete. When Emily, the night unit's bully, closed in on her one evening, demanding to know why the chart rack was a mess, Susan had a meltdown. Even though this was not Susan's responsibility, she found herself literally backed against the wall in the locker room as Emily went on a tirade about how Susan was always running late and never finished her work.

When Emily walked away with a self-satisfied smile, a few of her coworkers looked at each other in amusement as they finished preparing for work. Not one of them reached out to Susan. Although Susan made it as far as the parking lot without crying, she couldn't prevent the tears from rolling down her cheeks once she reached her car. In between sobs, she called Mia, her closest friend and coworker, to describe what had just happened. Although they resolved to tell their supervisor about Emily, who had been treating both of them like naughty children for many months, in the end, neither of them wanted to cause problems. They continued to complain to each other but said nothing to anyone else.

The Bystander

There's an extremely large group of nurses who are often overlooked in the RA dynamic. They're called bystanders. Almost everyone has been in this role at one time or another. (Think back on my early relationship with Janet.)

In its simplest form, a bystander is just what it sounds like: someone who stands by and watches while others are abused. She may snicker or stare dead-faced, but she doesn't walk away, which is important. The bully often draws her power from these witnesses, which is an important cue to interventions we'll discuss later.

Bystanders are often uncomfortable seeing someone else be the victim of RA, because it's pretty likely we've all been in the victim's position at one time or another. One nurse told me of an incident when she was charting in a corner while another group of nurses gossiped about a colleague, unaware of her presence. She sat and listened, wishing she had the courage to stand up and tell them to stop. "I couldn't do it," she confessed, "but I left that night wondering if they were talking about me, since I was a known friend of their previous target. I should have done something."

I should have done something when I was Janet's un-willing sidekick, too, but I was afraid of this much-older nurse who seemed to know everything about our profession that would help me succeed. If I didn't have her help, how would I make it as a nurse? (It turned out there were lots of other people just as knowledgeable and willing to support me.)

Sometimes, though, bystanders are all too willing to be part of the action. They form a posse around the bully or actively scope out new targets for her aggression. Other bystanders may just stand and titter while the bully lets loose on her victim. If asked, they will tell you they aren't involved in relational aggression because their behavior isn't aggressive or demeaning. It was all the bully nurse's fault. Think again.

Where Does Aggression Come From?

Every man and woman on this earth has probably been too aggressive at some point in their life, whether it was fighting with a sibling, saying something mean to a boyfriend or girlfriend, or blowing off steam at a coworker who happened to walk up to their desk with the latest annual report on company recycling policies. It's a terrible feeling to say something cruel or mean to a person who doesn't deserve it; the minute the words are out of your mouth, you regret them.

This type of aggression is not what I'm describing when I refer to a nurse who operates in RA mode 24/7. This nurse is on the lookout for victims (who she may in fact view as potential threats) at the gym, in her community, and at work. In high school, she probably operated much the same way as she does now, thinking she was getting what she wanted. Perhaps she did, but not because people liked her. The reality is that people do her bidding because they're afraid of her.

The classic "queen bee" aggressor was Joan Crawford, who, in a 1955 movie of the same name (*Queen Bee*) played a woman whose behavior ranged from sweetly vicious to openly cruel. Thus, a stereotype was born that captured the subtle but extremely negative behaviors women use to hurt each other. The exaggerated sigh or toss of one's hair, the mocking voice, and the denigrating rumors are all weapons of choice. No one knows for sure why females tend toward more covert behaviors to express aggression, while males are more likely to use physical forms of conflict, but there are different theories.

Powerlessness

Perhaps a sense of overt powerlessness leads to more subtle struggles through aggressive behavior. Attridge (1996) discusses the lack of power that nurses have had in making positive changes in their work environment, which leads to frustration and job dissatisfaction. Manojlovich (2007) concurs, noting that powerless nurses are ineffective nurses, and goes on to elaborate on the psychological consequences of this condition. In many ways, feeling a sense of powerlessness shapes a nurse's approach to his or her work and colleagues.

On the other hand, Boudrias, Gaudreau, and Laschinger (2004) suggest that when workers feel empowered, they are more likely to take an active role in shaping their work environment in a positive way. Chandler (1992) takes the concept of empowerment one step further by examining it from a social feminist perspective. According to her and to others (Fletcher et al., 2006; Wuest, 1994), women do not gain a sense of power from having equal status to men or enhanced decision making, but rather through emotional growth and nurturing relationships. Perhaps this is why in high-stress environments like hospitals, where there may be no sense of cooperation, nurses who feel little connection to each other are prone to relational aggression.

Evolutionary Biology

The theory of evolutionary biology and psychology posits a different view. Researchers such as Campbell (1993) and Barash and Lipton (2002) believe that women are not by nature aggressive, but that this behavior occurs as a protective measure. Women learn to make sure their children will survive by defeating other women in order to win a good partner who will take care of them and provide resources. However, women need the same women they compete with for male protectors to help them survive pregnancy and child-rearing when men are away foraging and hunting. Thus, a paradoxical situation has existed throughout history: Women spend more time with each other in fairly limited quarters, while men are much freer to roam at a distance in small groups. Women are emotionally close and sensitive, but have the potential to be equally vicious and cruel.

Newer information on neurobiology from Louanne Brezendine (2006) makes a convincing case for the differences in hardwiring between male and female brains. According to Dr. Brezendine, while men are oriented toward independence, women get their self-esteem from relationships, which they try to maintain no matter the cost.

Neurochemical

Shelley Taylor, author of *The Tending Instinct,* suggests that the difference between male and female aggression is biochemical. While the well-known "fight or flight" response, activated largely by testosterone, is valid for males, females are disposed to "tend and befriend" through care-giving and attachment-type behaviors stimulated by oxytocin. Taylor and her colleagues go on to explain that covert forms of aggression are more common in women because women are more relational and cerebral in their expression.

Dunn (1999) reviews several studies that attest to differences in the way men and women communicate. For example, she shows that adult women are better than men at detecting nuances in nonverbal communication, just as girls both display and understand nurturing and nonverbal behavior better than boys do. It would make sense, then, that women would express their feelings of displeasure or conflict through negative, nonverbal behaviors. And perhaps nurses, the most nurturing of women, are among the quickest to interpret body language as a sign of approval or dismissal. Dunn points out that body language enhances the spoken message, especially for girls, who place greater emphasis on social relationships than boys do.

Sociocultural Context

Although relational aggression could be the result of communication styles, socialization also plays a role. This is the insight of Mary Pipher (1992), who was among the first to decry the "girl-poisoning" culture we live in. According to Pipher, the inability of girls (and therefore women) to find their own voice and speak out explains the higher incidence of psychosocial illnesses such as depression, eating disorders, cutting, etc., in females.

What Women Want

Regardless of the cause, Carol Gilligan and colleagues consider relationships pivotal for the development of psychological health in women. These researchers were pioneers in developing a psychology of women that wasn't just a knockoff version of male growth and development. They believe women achieve psychological milestones differently than men, and that relationships are key to their growth (Gilligan, 1993).

Other authors suggest that the cultural conditioning that encourages women to suppress anger and allows men to have all the power is at the root of relational aggression. Inevitably, women learn other ways to express their negative emotions, but the behaviors are so nuanced that only another woman will understand them.

Regardless of which theory is right, it's clear that relationally aggressive behaviors are more prevalent in women. They are often driven by a sense of threat or fear and are motivated internally. They are also behaviors that can, like most behaviors, be changed.

Exercise

Think of times throughout your life when you experienced conflict with another woman. How did you resolve the situation as: a child, a teenager, a young adult, and a mature woman? Is there a pattern in your relationship style that supports the theories in this chapter—feeling powerless, the belief that women don't express anger, or some other?

Has your relationship style changed over the years? Would you like it to? List what you consider your strengths and weaknesses and compare with those of a person you admire.

5 | victimology

The most obvious and classic victim of RN RA has always been the student nurse. Having taught in several different nursing programs, the constant I've seen in nursing education is the treatment of nursing students in the same way I'm told some physicians "teach" medical students: by humiliating and demeaning them. When I was an instructor, most of the mistreatment came from nurses who worked in the hospitals and agencies where students obtained their clinical experience, but some of it came from the educators themselves. I'm not talking about teachers who had high standards for patient care and stuck to them, or instructors who expected professional behavior as part of nursing education. I'm talking about individuals who used behaviors on the list in Chapter 3 to "educate."

Not So New

While the new nurse may be, literally, fresh out of school, he or she may also be experienced, but new to a particular hospital or geographic location. Vessey et al. (2009) found that those nurses who had been employed fewer than five years on a unit were more likely to be treated with relational aggression than those who had been there longer. Consider the following, which was shared with me by a nurse who found herself unwillingly cast in the victim role. There were also plenty of bystanders who watched as she was abused.

Rita was the first nurse practitioner to be hired at a nursing home in a suburb near the city where she had completed her graduate degree. She was also the first nurse of color to work at the facility, which the physician who recruited her said would not be a problem. He thought highly of Rita, who had been precepted by one of his colleagues, and established a routine in which she made rounds at the nursing home where he was medical director and followed protocols they had established to address problems. He had paved the way for her presence by informing Linda, the director of nursing, an RN with an associate degree who had worked at the nursing home for 20 years, that Rita would be visiting in his place at the nursing home every other day.

Rita says she could tell from the minute she arrived that Linda was not happy to have her at the nursing home, and her behavior influenced the rest of the staff. Before long, Rita was refused access to charts when she needed them, made to wait for staff to give her updates on patients, and treated rudely. She learned of a rumor circulating that she was incompetent and had been fired from her previous job.

At first, Rita fought back by trying to win the staff over. She was good-natured and even helped them out with a resident's care here and there. After talking with the physician who hired her, she thought things would get better, but they didn't.

"I couldn't figure out if it was because of my role, which threatened Linda, or my skin color, which was obviously new to the entire institution," she says. "There were a few auxiliary staff who were of color, but none of the aides or nurses."

Rita ended up leaving the job and even considered filing a lawsuit against the nursing home. Her physical health suffered along with her emotional well-being (or lack thereof). Worst of all was the lack of confidence and shame she felt after the treatment she had received. What if Linda was right? What if Rita really was a bad nurse practitioner and didn't know what she was doing?

Emotional Fallout

Most victims share Rita's feelings, and that's where the pain of relational aggression comes in. As victims wonder, "Why me?" a little voice inside their heads whispers an answer: "Maybe it's true. Maybe everyone you work with doesn't like you." Over and over again, I hear victims ask for an explanation as to why they were selected as targets. All too often, however, the reason lies inside the aggressor and may never be known. That doesn't prevent the sense of betrayal, shame, and hurt that victims feel. It's maddening, especially when the aggression is prolonged or part of a campaign, as happened with Rita.

When I was thrust into the world of full-time nursing and worked in high-acuity hospitals, I saw how another nurse could protect your back and help you finish your work on time. I also knew that same nurse could have a bad day and rip you to shreds with her words or behavior. When I worked as an agency nurse in Philadelphia and traveled from hospital to hospital, I saw the same relational behaviors happen again and again. Although students or younger nurses often took the brunt of the permanent nurses' hostility, frequently for unknown reasons, anyone could be a target.

As an instructor, when I went to nursing homes on my practice days, I was met with mixed responses. To be honest, most of the nurses were thrilled to have someone who would take the time to answer their questions and sit with patients for as long as needed. But there were some who questioned why I was there and refused to help me find supplies or needed information. In the early days of integrating the advanced-practice role into clinics, hospitals and other organizations, it wasn't unusual to get the cold shoulder from RNs already employed there. Now that the concept of advanced-practice nurses has been accepted and relationships within the health care team are much better, RA seems to be less of a problem. Still, when it does happen, it is baffling to have members of your own profession turn on you because you went the extra step and returned to school for further education.

Crabs in a Pot

According to the theory of oppressed groups (Fanon, 1963; Freire, 2000), people who are dominated by others turn on each other and become self-deprecating because they have internalized the values of the group in control. These beliefs underlie the concept of horizontal violence, which posits that women keep each other down, believing if a person succeeds, it's bad for the group, and that there's limited space "at the top." Therefore, when those in an oppressed group encounter others who are bettering themselves through education or some other means, they feel resentment and envy instead of encouragement. While it sounds like an explanation, that's not what happened to Emily.

"I was pregnant with my first child after working on the same unit for three years," she recalls. "I admit I was fortunate, but I made the mistake of telling another nurse who asked that I was going to be able to pursue my graduate degree after I had the baby while my mother-in-law babysat. I didn't think I said it in a bragging way or even an excited way; I was just factual. But soon a few nurses on the unit started treating me like dirt, refusing to help me with patients and even not speaking to me. When others held a surprise baby shower for me, these nurses didn't attend or even say goodbye on my last day of work."

If you've been a victim, like Emily, you inevitably ask the question, "What did I do wrong?" It hurt her to think her behavior may have triggered another nurse to be mean or rude, and although the majority of nurses on her unit were warm and supportive, those few who weren't are the ones Emily remembers now, years later.

Aggression-Proof

Victims can be found anywhere and at any level of nursing. Supervisors can be victims of vicious behavior from nurse managers. ("Well, if you just did a better job on your end, my unit wouldn't be such a mess," or "You're the one who decides on all the policies—why blame me when they don't work out?") Unit clerks can be vicious to nurses; nurses can abuse medical students; and even nursing students can harass and demean their instructors.

The danger, of course, is that once you are treated like a victim, you begin to believe the comments are true. With each cruel word, a bit of your self-confidence leaks away until there's not much left. Eventually, you appear to be that worn-down nurse who doesn't have much going for her. Some nurses say that after a while, the victim role spills over into other domains of their lives, and they unconsciously seek out friends and romantic partners who treat them in much the same way as their original aggressors.

The most unfortunate part of this story is, of course, that it's not true. Aggressors thrive on making others feel bad about themselves, which can only happen if a victim believes that what she's being told is true. Consider this: If the aggressor/bully had never entered your life, you wouldn't have thought about the negative things she accused you of. So what makes them true now?

Exercise

Have you ever been or have you ever seen a nurse who was the victim of someone's RA? How did it affect you/her in these ways:

- Physically

- Mentally

- Professionally

- With friends

- With your/her spouse or romantic partner

- With family

What could you/she do to step out of the victim role?

6 | bystanders

Not every nurse is an aggressor or target. In fact, most fall into a larger, third group: bystanders. Bystanders can take on a variety of roles. They might be a facilitator of aggression—too timid to actually start anything hostile, but willing to encourage someone else's aggression by laughing or being part of the rumor chain. Or they may be silent observers, uncomfortable with what is happening but unsure of how to intervene to stop things.

Not Actively Aggressing

Franny found out about the power of bystanders when several of her coworkers seemed to snicker every time she walked into the nurses' station. Since this was relatively new behavior on their part, she tried to figure out what she could have done to incur their ridicule.

"Have you noticed anything different about the way I've been treated lately?" she asked her charge nurse, Alyse, who shrugged her shoulders.

"It's just a bunch of women acting like juveniles. Don't let it get you down," Alyse said. "You're doing fine as far as I'm concerned, so whatever has their feathers ruffled is no big deal."

But it *was* a big deal, especially when Franny overheard Trish, the most outspoken of those who were taunting her, talking to a group of other nurses around the corner of a hallway. "Franny'll find out he only goes after sluts," Trish said. "Remember what happened to Ginny? She quit the NICU after they broke up." There were twitters of agreement and amusement in response to her declaration.

Franny was so dumbstruck by the talk, she forgot that Trish usually intimidated her. With her hands on her hips, she turned the corner and faced a group of five nurses—Trish and four of her followers. "I don't know who you think is chasing after me," said Franny. "But I'll have you know my boyfriend has nothing to do with this place. I learned a long time ago never to mix business and pleasure."

Stalking away from the stunned crowd, Franny suddenly realized that they were referring to one of the attending physicians who had graduated from the same college as she. They had known each other distantly while undergraduates, but now, having relocated in a big city, they had connected as friends and sometimes ate lunch together. The idea of a romantic relationship between them was actually funny. From that point on, Franny stopped caring about the gossiping posse of her coworkers.

If Franny had had less confidence, being singled out by Trish and having other nurses fail to stand up for her would have bothered her more each day, especially when others joined in on the harassment. The other nurses who took part in the put-down made it seem all the more likely to be true—at least somewhat. And even if no one believed there was a romance going on, they must have disliked Franny enough to join Trish's hostility toward her, right? In any case, although Franny's indifference to their taunts disarmed Trish and her followers, it wasn't long before they found another less strong victim.

Why Worry About Bystanders?

Bystanders are an interesting group. Sometimes they follow an aggressor because they long for acceptance, even if it means doing something hurtful to another person. Other times, bystanders are afraid that if they aren't aligned with the aggressor, they may become the next target, so their "follow the leader" style of bullying is a form of self-defense.

Not every bystander is quite so consciously cruel. In fact, if you work on a unit or in an organization where RA is rampant, you may be forced into the role of bystander whether you like it or not. Every day when you go to work, you'll be immersed in a toxic environment created by conflicts you have no part in but can't help witnessing. In many ways, patients are also bystanders to this kind of tension, and can pick up on relationship problems between coworkers just by observation.

Bystanders can take on a variety of roles: actively abetting the aggressor, passively serving as a conduit for RA, watching in righteous indignation as someone else "gets what they deserve," or standing by uncomfortably, not knowing how to help and fearing they will be the next victim.

What's Your Bystander-Ability?

If you're not sure where you fall on the bystander continuum, ask yourself these questions:

1. If someone tells me potentially damaging information about a coworker, I would:

    A. Keep it to myself.

    B. Ask another nurse if she thinks it's true.

    C. Tell the target of the rumor that she really needs to know what people are saying about her.

2. When there's a controversy between coworkers, I usually find myself:

   A. Trying to keep track of what's going on with each side so I can avoid conflict.

   B. Siding with whomever has the most power on my unit or organization.

   C. Avoiding the situation completely, even when others try to involve me.

3. If a "queen bee" nurse berates a new intern, I am likely to:

   A. Walk away and feel bad for the new nurse.

   B. Watch to see how the new nurse will respond.

   C. Tell the "queen bee" nurse to remember when she was a newbie and go easy on the intern.

4. If one of my coworkers told me she was ready to tell off a "queen bee" unit secretary who makes life miserable for everyone, I would:

   A. Tell my coworker that the secretary is divorced and filed for bankruptcy not long ago, which is why she's so crabby to everyone.

   B. Go to the unit manager and tell her she has a big problem because of the secretary.

C. Tell my coworker I agree with her, but suggest we try to do something other than gang up on the secretary to resolve the problem.

5. I am the nurse on my unit who everyone comes to with gossip. When this happens, I:

A. Tell some of my coworkers what I've heard, but not others.

B. Wonder why people choose to come to me with such stories.

C. Share the gossip with the unit manager so she can take action against the person it's about.

If you picked these answers—1: A, 2: C, 3: A, 4: C, and 5: B—then good for you. You are the most benign bystander and avoid getting actively involved in RA. As in reality, the bystander can be the most influential person in the bullying dynamic. All it takes to defuse a lot of RA is for a group of nurses who belong to the "queen bee" clique to walk away and leave their aggressive leader without a hive of supporter bees. Or, if a bystander decides to intervene, as happened in answer C for question 3, she's suddenly a hero. While adult aggressors rely less on the support and approval of others, they will think twice about persisting when enough bystanders ask them to stop.

Exercise

Think of alternatives to bystander behavior that you feel comfortable with:

- Walking away from a nurse using RA to hurt another.

- Confronting the aggressor about her behavior—either at the time it occurs or later.

- Talking with the victim and telling her you disagree.

List any others and next time you find yourself in a bystander role, see if you can try them out.

7 | some nurses are better than others—really?

Most of the literature written about nurses being bullied implies that someone in a superior position uses behavior that is relationally aggressive to bully and hurt his or her subordinate. While "bosses" (and nurses seem to have many, from their shift supervisor all the way up to the director or CEO of nursing) may intimidate by the innate power they hold, other coworkers can be relationally aggressive, too. The terms "horizontal" or "lateral violence" don't quite capture the kind of aggression that occurs among nurses. A coworker doesn't have to be superior to you to have the power to hurt you; she just has to display the behavior that makes you feel insufficient.

"I'll never forget Cassie," one nurse said. "She was the nastiest unit secretary we ever had. If you got on her wrong side, she would take her time putting your charts together or paging doctors when you asked her to. Even our charge nurse couldn't handle her. I was so happy when she retired!"

Then there are support staff, who often have more responsibility than they're prepared for. Not all their negligent behavior is deliberate, but when they form a clique and band together against another worker, the results can be not only damaging, but also disastrous.

"I remember Lucille," Nan shudders. "She was about a foot taller than me and a lot heavier. She kept muttering under her breath about 'new graduates who think they know everything.' When I checked the vital-signs sheet, one of our post-op patients had spiked a fever and she hadn't even bothered to tell me! By the time I found out, the man was really sick. That was just one of many mishaps."

Nan felt powerless because Lucille was part of a group of unionized workers whom she feared. The next day, when she told the charge nurse about the situation, she was asked to write up an incident report, which only made Lucille's abuse worse. Over time, Nan stuck to her guns, and eventually Lucille backed off when she realized she wasn't going to ruffle Nan. But nurses on other floors reported their displeasure at having to work for Lucille when she was pulled to their units. Eventually, Lucille crossed the line one too many times and caused one too many errors with her poor communication skills. As a consequence, she was fired.

Intergenerational Relationships

It seems to be an unspoken rite of passage to mistreat new graduates, who come to work eager to apply all the knowledge they have amassed in their education. Today, for the first time in history, as many as four different generations of nurses may be working closely together, each with their own sets of values, attitudes, expectations, and motivations. Olson (2008) offers an excellent overview of these generations and how contextual conflicts may arise among them. A summary of her descriptions follows:

- **Matures:** Matures, who are 60 and over, may operate from a framework of more traditional values, such as loyalty to an institution and the people in it, automatic respect for people in positions of authority, obedience to rules (even if they don't make sense), and the belief that hard work is part of the job.

- **Baby boomers:** Baby boomers (about 44 to 62 years old) are a large group with values similar to matures, but also oriented toward competition and success, which is often reflected by salary and status. Having come of age in an era when women began to enter the workforce, baby boomers may be the first to regard nursing as a career rather than just a job.

- **Generation Xers:** Generation Xers (25 to 45 years old) are more likely to be independent and motivated by things that satisfy them, rather than by loyalty. For example, Gen Xers likely won't automatically respect authority or unquestioningly accept rules. They also are techno-savvy and oriented toward personal goals. A study by Leiter (2011) demonstrated that nurses aged 30 to 48, whom he called Gen Xers, were more dissatisfied at work and reported more bullying.

- **Millennials:** Also referred to as Generation Y, these individuals, described as the "me generation," are younger than age 29. Their parents are most likely baby boomers. This group is diverse and globally oriented, multitasks, and views work as a way to earn money to satisfy their needs.

Given such a mix of characteristics, clashes between new nurses (who may hail from the millennial generation) and mature nurses (who have completely different attitudes toward work) seem inevitable. Intergenerational differences can exacerbate preexisting tendencies to "put new nurses through their paces," or orient them using the "trial-by-fire" method many older nurses experienced when beginning their first jobs.

"I'll never forget Audra," said Marci, a baby boomer charge nurse who had worked on the same unit for three years. "One time, she got her assignment and came up to me with her hand on her hip and this sour look on her face. 'You expect me to do all this?' she asked, right in my face. It was all I could do to keep my cool and tell her 'I sure do.' She flounced away, and I could see the tattoo on the back of her neck. At least it was small, but the policy was to keep them covered."

Culture and Ethnicity

Cultural diversity is another factor that influences not only the patients we care for, but the nursing workforce. Discrimination and RA are not new behaviors. "As an African-American woman in the health care industry, I have no other choice. Regrettably, I face racism from every corner—from white colleagues and even from my own people," wrote Gloria Ramsey (Finkelstein, 1997, p. 21) in a book of stories about nurses' first year of work. She recalls watching television with white students in nursing school and being offended by demeaning portrayals of minorities. When she spoke up, her classmates ridiculed her and acted as if she was being unreasonable. Throughout her 22 years as a nurse, RA from nurses of all ethnicities has continued for Ramsey, who notes, "Racism from your own people is more pathetic" (p. 22).

As nurses from other countries become part of organizations and hospitals where traditions are longstanding, it can be difficult for both groups to understand each other. This happened to Flora, an RN who was a new hire on a medical-surgical floor. Flora escaped the usual difficulties of new nurses because she was such a hard worker. Whenever someone was needed to work a double, Flora volunteered. While her coworkers clustered their days off around the December holidays, Flora took a minimum of time off.

When summer came, however, that changed. The July schedule had barely been posted when an angry buzz traveled from one nurse to the other. Flora had the entire month of July off! Before they could deluge Flora with demands for an explanation, Mandy, the head nurse, called an impromptu meeting. She walked the nurses through the past year and showed them how many extra days Flora had worked. "But that's not what's most important," Mandy said, turning to Flora.

"In my country," explained Flora, "we all come together in July so my children can see their relatives. Everyone is too poor to fly to the United States, so we have to go to them. It's the only time we can be together." Mandy finished by saying, "When I hired Flora, I made an arrangement to let her use all her days off in July."

There was an uncomfortable silence, and then the nurses drifted away from the station. No one mentioned

Flora's vacation again. In fact, when the time came for her to leave, a few nurses even wished her a good time.

Flowers (2004) identifies five components of cultural competence for nurses:

- Awareness of one's own cultural beliefs, especially those that might influence your interactions with groups of clients or nurses who are different from you

- Questioning how much you know about the different cultural groups you come into contact with, especially as it relates to health and illness

- Identifying culturally important information that influences your perception of clients and nurses who come from backgrounds different from yours

- Being direct in asking questions and seeking to understand beliefs and practices that are culturally based but that you may not understand

- Seeking to learn more about other cultural backgrounds—and not waiting to do so until you are forced to because of an issue or difficult situation

Had the nurses on Flora's unit taken the time to consider these cultural competencies, their relationships with Flora might not have suffered. It took a long time for the strain of their "righteous" anger to wear off.

Other situations occur when nurses from other countries don't assimilate or attempt to join the rest of the team, staying in their own cliques, speaking in their native tongue, and shutting others out. "They're like the girls in high school who all spoke Spanish and used it to gossip about us so we wouldn't understand," Ann explains. She works at a large urban hospital where many nurses who don't speak English as their first language resort to their native tongue when not providing patient care. Oftentimes, she and her coworkers are offended by coworkers who cluster together and shut others out by speaking in a different language.

Males, RA, and Nursing

Although the phenomenon of men entering the nursing profession may seem novel, this is only because most history books focus on women (O'Lynn and Tranbarger, 2007). Historically, medics in the military, religious orders devoted to healing the sick, and several non-military nursing orders were entirely male. It wasn't until Florence Nightingale came along that the gender mix changed, shaping the nursing field into a female-dominated profession.

The differences in relationships between males and females also involve behavioral differences, such as changes in the communication style. For example, Yoshimura and

Hayden (2007) and Tannen (1994) note several differences between the way males and females interact, which may have an impact on nursing.

Male-Female Talk Patterns

	Content of Communication	Nature of Communication	Verbal/ Nonverbal	Expectations	Downtime
Females	Information sharing, rapport talk	Relational	Body language part of message	Expects to receive feedback	Small talk, friendly talk
Males	Goal-directed	Informational	Verbal	Expects to receive feedback only if there are problems	Extraneous talk not essential

In addition to communication differences, there may be tensions at work between male and female nurses because of territoriality. Women may not welcome men into what they perceive as a women's profession. Indeed, male nurses have commented that they are sometimes made to feel like intruders.

"Guys would never do that to each other, but with women, it was like, why would you want to be here? What's wrong with you?" Mike, an ED nurse said, recalling his first job. In addition to the RA that came his way, he saw the nurses attacking each other with equal ferocity.

"I always had to do twice as much, twice as well," Clark, a medical supply company administrator explained. "So I finally left and went into another field where I could use my nursing skills but didn't have to work with just women. As soon as I left, everything changed. I was so much happier at my new job where it was an equal mix of men and women and not just nurses."

At the same time, nurses complain that men are more likely to obtain preferred positions because of their gender. Hader (2010) surveyed 1,500 nurse leaders and found that male nurses move into management positions at younger ages than women and earn higher salaries than women do. But it's not all rosy for men; Crawford (2009) found that male nurses were abused by patients nearly 10 percent more often.

Exercise

How diverse is the unit where you work? Is there a mix of ages and ethnicities? How have differences in beliefs and values related to different cultural or generational backgrounds led to RA? Have you ever been ridiculed or teased because of a belief or value that is important to you but not to anyone else? What options do you have when this happens?

II | healing from the inside out

8 | a crash course in RA recovery

Maybe you've read to this point and feel as if none of the information in this book relates to you. You enjoy your coworkers, and for the most part, the relationships between the people with whom you interact on a day-to-day basis are respectful and rewarding. If that's the case, you won't need to go much further (unless you're trying to help someone else or you've bought this book as a gift for a troubled friend).

Even so, humor me. Try answering the following questions and ask yourself how involved you *really* are on the RA continuum, realizing that it's often hard to have insight into our own behavior. Janice, a "queen bee" graduate student I once taught, described herself as "driven." Similarly, a friend of mine works with a nurse she describes as classic manipulator, but that person says she's a "people person" who knows how to "get results." Little do these women know that everyone else considers them to be female bullies.

RA Quotient

Not sure how you might score on the RA scale? Consider the statements below. (Obviously, the more "Yes" answers you accumulate, the more RA plays a role in your everyday life. For a reproducible copy of these questions, see Appendix A, "RA Quotient.")

1. I've changed jobs a lot because of the people I had to work with.

   _____ Yes   _____ No

2. I've left a job before my orientation period was finished because I knew I wouldn't get along with the nurses on the unit where I would be working.

   _____ Yes   _____ No

3. Every day, on my way to work, I feel myself becoming physically stressed because I don't want to go there.

   _____ Yes   _____ No

4. If another nurse does something rude or mean to me, I plan what I will say or do to get even with her and strike when the opportunity presents itself.

   _____ Yes   _____ No

5. I'm always angry when I'm at work, but I rarely tell anyone.

_____ Yes   _____ No

6. I'm sick of watching the other people on my unit bicker.

_____ Yes   _____ No

7. People I work with don't like me, and I don't care. None of them are worth hanging around with anyway.

_____ Yes   _____ No

8. I take secret joy in seeing another coworker get what she deserves for poor performance.

_____ Yes   _____ No

9. My nurse manager/supervisor promotes relational aggression and bullying on our unit by playing favorites and creating drama.

_____ Yes   _____ No

10. Secretly, I think I am more competent than most of the people I work with. It's a shame.

_____ Yes   _____ No

11. Having good relationships among coworkers is important to the administration of my hospital/organization.

_____ Yes   _____ No

12. I work harder than everyone else on my unit.

    _____ Yes   _____ No

13. No one gets the last word with me. Even if I have to respond later, I'll make sure they know I can't be pushed around.

    _____ Yes   _____ No

14. At least once a day when I'm at work I listen to gossip, pass on gossip, start gossip, or am the subject of gossip.

    _____ Yes   _____ No

15. If I'm angry, I sometimes ignore or act rude to my coworkers as a stress reliever.

    _____ Yes   _____ No

16. I get excluded from joining others in breaks or meals, or I do the excluding.

    _____ Yes   _____ No

17. The emotional climate at my workplace is toxic because of the nurses who work there.

    _____ Yes   _____ No

18. My feelings are often hurt by people/women I work with.

    _____ Yes   _____ No

19. I can't say no to my coworkers without worrying they will be upset with me.

   _____ Yes   _____ No

20. When I see other nurses being bullied, I feel bad. But I don't want to get involved, so I say nothing.

   _____ Yes   _____ No

After you answer these questions and have a sense of the impact of RA on your everyday work life, think about your current job satisfaction. If you can, try to determine what makes you feel the way you do about the place where you work. Here are a few possibilities:

- Salary

- Work responsibilities

- Coworkers

- Supervisors

- Location of workplace/commute

- Work hours

- Boredom

- Emotional environment/RA

Your History of Satisfaction

Next, take a few minutes and reflect on your nursing career. If you have a résumé handy, pull it out. Rate each of the jobs you've had on a scale of 1 to 10, with 10 being "best," and 1 being "worst." Identify your favorite job (hopefully you had one) and break down the components that made it enjoyable. Was it the type of nursing you were doing? Or perhaps your coworkers made the position enjoyable. Did a special sense of teamwork or unity make you glad to be part of that particular organization?

Compare the answers to those questions with how you feel about the job you have right now. You may already be on your way to understanding what tangible things need to change—if any—in order for you to change your behavior. For example, if you feel you aren't being paid adequately, there are steps you can take to try to remedy that situation. Your attempts to adjust your income might not be successful, but you'll at least gain some helpful knowledge. Your feelings about being unfairly compensated could well lead you to interact with your coworkers in ways that have nothing to do with your real feelings about them—or vice versa. Taking the time to pinpoint the source of your job satisfaction or dissatisfaction provides you with a healthy insight that could be what's blocking your ability to feel positive about your work life.

The Importance of Self-Esteem

Another important assessment is your professional self-esteem. Similar to your personal self-esteem, your professional self-esteem will influence your behavior in ways you may be completely unaware of. If you feel like the least talented nurse at your workplace and constantly need to prove your worth, of course you'll be defensive about feedback on your performance. Alternatively, you may take a proactive stance and lash out at others before they can pick up on your deficits. Alternatively, you might not feel challenged enough in your current position, so boredom brings you down every day.

To get a sense of how you feel about your abilities, do the 1–10 test again, giving yourself a score for each of the following items. As before, 1 will be worst, and 10 will be best.

_____ *I feel I have reached the nursing goals I set for myself.*

_____ *I am recognized for my achievements at work.*

_____ *I work well with my coworkers and trust them.*

_____ *My coworkers would say they work well with me and trust me.*

_____ *I have confidence in my ability to do my current job.*

_____ *I am as productive as the other nurses I work with.*

_____ *I hold myself accountable for my nursing assignments.*

_____ *My colleagues would describe my nursing abilities in a positive way.*

Add up your score to determine where you rank. Higher scores indicate a higher professional self-esteem. If your score is low, maybe what's really bothering you about your current job is not your difficult coworkers, but your own feelings about work. Perhaps it's time to try something new or ask your supervisor for some feedback on your nursing strengths.

The Importance of Communication

Although we all think we know how to get a message across, it's not as simple as talking and listening. For example, one person saying, "I *like* your haircut," while smiling, gives a different message than the person who says, "I like your *haircut*," with her voice becoming progressively lower as her eyebrows become progressively higher. Effective communication is a "win-win" situation where both parties feel heard and respected. No one interrupts, shouts, or bullies the other during the talk.

Body language is another aspect of communication that is particularly important for women (Dellasega, 2004). We often "read" into another woman's message based on her posture, facial expression, eye contact, and so on. Many times, our impressions of another woman are formed with our first sight of her, before she utters a word. Naomi Wolf's classic text showed that beautiful women have the hardest time being accepted and respected by their own gender (1991).

Unfortunately, being treated as a victim early in life can turn one into a backlash bully, or it can become a self-fulfilling role that is hard to leave behind. It can also affect how you communicate as an adult. Consider Mary, a lifelong victim who has trouble looking people in the eye when they speak and barely whispers when she talks. Mary is tentative when approaching doctors and placating patients. In contrast, her coworker Lola is assertive but not aggressive, holding eye contact and nodding to indicate she understands what's being said. When Lola speaks, her voice is confident and her words thoughtful. It's not coincidental that Lola wasn't caught up in RA as a girl, and often stood up for girls who were being bullied.

However, there's a huge difference between assertive and aggressive communication, and not many people understand it, let alone put it into practice. Nurses, like many other professionals, receive little education on how to communicate with each other or with patients and administrators in a way that leaves both parties feeling as if they've been "heard."

Aggressive Versus Assertive Communication

	Woman One	Woman Two
Aggressive	I win	You lose
Passive	I lose	You win
Assertive	I win	You win

Listening Skills

At the same time, listening skills help promote clear and productive communication. Looking directly at the person who is speaking, giving him or her your full attention, and rephrasing your understanding of what he or she said are just a few ways to promote effective communication.

In today's complex hospital environment, effective communication is vital to safe patient care (Manojlovich & DeCicco, 2007). Several studies concerning physician bullying of nurses linked this dysfunction to patient care errors (Aleccia, 2008), but nurse-to-nurse communication is equally important. When one nurse relates to another with the intent of humiliating, manipulating, intimidating, or otherwise bullying him or her, it's likely that the content of the conversation will be a secondary focus.

Vessey et al. (2009) reviewed several studies that, if taken as a whole, support the adverse effects of relational aggression on patient care, job satisfaction, patient outcomes, and absenteeism.

Gossip is a particularly negative communication style. It can undermine any nursing unit. Women in particular seem to be prone to seeking out a spicy story, embellishing it, and passing it along. In fact, Nicholson (2001)found that others are more likely to respond to negative information about someone they don't know than to positive information. That's probably because the gossiper is giving you the impression that he or she trusts you enough to share particularly vital information with you. Alternatively, it could be a test of your loyalty.

Plus, as one nurse, Norma, confessed: "Who wants to hear that Jeremy is a great nurse? It's much more interesting to know he's dating the female chief resident of dermatology, who's a stunner." Seems harmless enough, right? But what if Jeremy is married or engaged to someone else and that person hears the rumor? Or, how about the resident? Would she be happy to know her love life was top news on the hospital hotline? Gossip may seem simple and harmless, but it always has the potential to hurt someone. So next time someone comes to you with a saucy tidbit of information, before passing it along to others, ask yourself:

- Do I know for sure that it's true?

- Will sharing this help someone?

- Would I repeat it if the subject of the gossip was here?

- What is my motivation for telling others what I have heard?

Make Your Work Life Better

All too often, we go through our daily routines without much awareness of our behavior. In many ways, it's an adaptive mechanism; without it, we'd have to figure out how to do our job anew each day. The problem with this, though, is that we can slide into behaviors that aren't healthy for us or for those around us. Eventually, those behaviors become who we are. Unless you receive a pretty intense wake-up call, you won't do much to change your way of being.

If you ask an aggressor why she treats her coworkers so shabbily, chances are she'll be shocked to hear you suggest that she does such a thing. She might describe herself as a nurse who has high standards and expects no less of others, but a bully? Not her!

In the same way, if you ask the perennial target why she lets others treat her with so little respect, she'll probably wrinkle her forehead in confusion. Her? Being taken advantage of because she gets manipulated into finishing up for other nurses every day, making her consistently late to leave? Never!

Why We Do the Things We Do

It's always important to think about what motivates behavior, be it yours, a patient's, or the foul-mouthed resident who makes it her mission to torment nurses. Maslow's Hierarchy of Needs, from your basic psychology class, proposed that all behavior is structured around a variety of needs. Until the lowest needs are met, you cannot think about higher-order ones. So, if you are not healthy, are not well-fed, and don't feel safe in your environment, you are unlikely to be thinking about whether your current job is fulfilling enough to be the career you want to pursue for the rest of your life.

I often think about this when I drive by the homeless people who cluster in our city square on cold winter mornings. Their lives operate on survival mode: many will come to the soup kitchen where I've volunteered for an hour of warmth and a filling meal, not to make new friends and have an interesting conversation with the volunteers. In the same way, a chronic master aggressor is struggling to protect her self-esteem and safety needs in every way she can think of. It's not likely she'll be reading a new book on being a better nurse in her off hours.

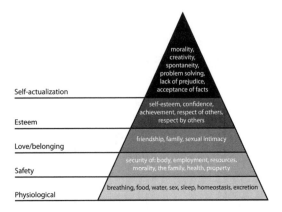

Maslow's Hierarchy of Needs

Understanding Motivations

So, when reflecting on your own behavior and trying to understand that of others, keep intrinsic motivation in mind. Think about what might be driving someone to act in ways that may seem, on the surface, to be irrational. Are there factors going on behind the scenes that you might not know about?

Next, think about what is driving *your* behavior. Are there things going on in your life that might be affecting your behavior? If you are planning a wedding, or you're worried about cutbacks at your spouse's job, or you didn't get much sleep the night before, chances are your behavior might not be the norm. You may be a bit grouchier than usual, less ready to volunteer for overtime, or not your usual patient self when a student nurse you are precepting can't seem to figure out how to give her first IM injection.

The "Won't Bee"

What about the nurses who won't be changed, no matter how hard you try? Consider what Kare Anderson, the "Say It Better Expert" (http://www.sayitbetter.com/), has to say about dealing with such individuals:

> *The most difficult woman in your life may have the most to teach you*
>
> *Bring out her good side*
>
> *Help her feel safe*
>
> *Find out what makes her feel happy or confident*
>
> *Make her look good*
>
> *Offer something*
>
> *Show good will to all*
>
> *Ask her: "Tell me more about that"*

Here are some other tactics that can help you defuse the overly aggressive nurse who has the entire unit feeling oppressed:

- **Figure out what makes her tick:** This takes you back to Maslow's Hierarchy of Needs or any number of subtle motivations embedded in it. If you know what's driving her behavior you might be able to address it. For example, if she gets cranky when she misses a meal, volunteer to get her lunch.

- **Understand what pushes her buttons:** Is she uneasy and likely to blow up at meetings? Or do shift changes freak her out? If so, can you soothe her and the people around her by thinning out crowds or trying to quiet the environment?

- **Be proactive:** Have a plan A, plan B, and plan C in place. Most aggressive nurses use the same tactics over and over again. Have several alternatives planned to deal with her. Maybe plan A is to walk away, plan B is to avoid being alone with her, and plan C is to discuss the situation with your unit manager.

- **Stake your boundaries and stick to them:** When you're out of the conflict, think about your bottom line ahead of time. What are you willing to do and not do?

- **Backlash aggression:** Beware of becoming an aggressor yourself! Sometimes, anger can build up to the point where you are in danger of exploding. Wait to confront your aggressor at some other time. Otherwise, a screaming match might occur.

- **Get outside help:** If it seems that you aren't going to be able to deal with a "won't bee" yourself, get outside help. Alternatively, explore procedures for filing a grievance.

It helps to make a concrete plan.

Not Sure What to Change?

Not sure what to change? This is a simple exercise that can help you get started. Get a journal and write out the following:

AWARE

A = Assess yourself and your relational style. *Think of whether you make friends easily and aren't troubled by social situations. You have lots of friends and rarely get into disagreements with them. Or are you easily intimidated by new people, sensing that they might be a threat to you? Is it hard for you to connect with other women socially, and do you go through a merry-go-round of gal pals, with a new "best friend" each week?*

W = What has gone on before? *Would others describe you as a good colleague and coworker?*

A = Awareness of choices, context, triggers. *What kinds of things might lead you to choose certain jobs or workplaces? What triggers might lead you to RA?*

R = Recognize relationship power. *Nurses united together have much more power than those who go it alone.*

E = Enforce, be accountable. *Think of ways to enforce your new behavior insights and make sure you follow them.*

These changes can mean that every day, someone can be blessed by your presence. You can be a change agent who helps others develop a vision of a better future. Don't stop with yourself, either! Never forget what happened on July 21, 2005, when 9,000 California nurses banded together, prompting then-Governor Arnold Schwarzenegger to back down on his intent to decrease the safe RN-to-patient staffing ratio from 1:5 to 1:6 (California Nurses Association, 2005). No single individual could have accomplished what the group was able to do together.

Inventorying Your RA

Think about some of your interactions with other women over the last 24 hours; then complete the chart below. Look for themes in feelings or behaviors that suggest you might be using an excess of aggressor, victim, or bystander behaviors. See the sample chart that follows for examples. Don't think too much about your answers until you've completed the exercise.

Your RA Inventory

The Place	The Person	The Behavior	What's Up With Me

For a reproducible copy of this inventory, see Appendix B, "Your RA Inventory."

Sample RA Inventory

The Place	The Person	The Behavior	What's Up With Me
Arrive at work, a little bit late	The new coworker	She asks me to look at a report she's working on. I blow her off because I don't have time.	Why does she try to get me to help her when it's obvious she wants my job? How dumb does she think I am?
My neighborhood	Next-door neighbor and walking crowd	They exclude me from walking with them—again. The leader of the pack hasn't been friendly since our kids had a fight shortly after we moved in.	What did I do wrong? I can't help it if our children don't get along.
Mother-in-law's house	Mother-in-law and sister-in-law	Both of them have been stay-at-home moms. They tell me about an article they just read on how bad day care is for children. Of course mine are in full-time, since I'm a nurse.	I'm sick and tired of the two of them suggesting they're supermoms and I'm the loser parent of the year.
Parenting website	Regular bloggers	A new mom posts a really stupid opinion about how anyone who uses disposable diapers is destroying the environment.	Like everyone else, I post about do-gooders who are ruining the economy.

From looking at this sample, it's clear to see that Jane, the author, had a negative mind-set in every domain of her life. She feels threatened by a colleague, paranoid about her neighbors, suspicious of her in-laws. She even gets involved in some cyber-bullying. While Jane doesn't list which behaviors she used in each situation, it doesn't take a stretch of the imagination to picture her giving the cold shoulder to her nurse orientee, making sure her neighbors know she's a runner, not a walker (and therefore better than them), and launching a verbal grenade at her in-laws. Her post about diapers is probably more vicious than factual. In the few minutes it's taken Jane to fill out this evaluation, her aggressive and bullying persona has emerged, even though she has probably never thought of herself as being anything but pleasant and straightforward with others.

Exercise

Create a plan for self-change at work. Begin with an RA behavior you want to work on immediately, and map out a strategy for eliminating it. For example, if you want to be more inclusive during lunchtime, commit to inviting a new nurse to join your crowd tomorrow. Track your behavior for a week and see how it goes, how you feel, and how others react.

Once you've worked on small changes, think about the big picture. Make a plan for behaviors that you would like to see changed in a month and in a year. Set goals for achieving this change. This exercise is especially powerful when you do it with a group and can hold each other accountable, but initially, trying out new behaviors on your own may be more comfortable.

9 | if no one's working together, it isn't a team

One of the hallmarks of health care is the high degree of teamwork involved. Ames et al. (1992) found that the more coworkers enjoyed and helped each other, the better their sense of being a team, and the higher their job satisfaction. Burnout and turnover is also lower among those teams where a sense of unity prevails (Shader et al., 2001).

Depending on the setting, there can be so many players involved that often the patient gets overlooked as the focus of care. Kim Dayton describes this poignantly in her story, "Procedures," which was published in *The Arduous Touch: Voices of Women in Health Care,* about women's experiences in health care (Haddad & Brown, 1999):

The nurse looked at the other one, the doctor, who was not really a doctor yet, and said, "Well, I think she will probably be here a long time."

Then the doctor, who was not really a doctor yet, said, "Have you gone down to the billing office?" And I said, "Yes, that's already taken care of." "Well, it says here that you need to be seen in billing, so perhaps you should go down there now." "But when will I get to see the baby?" And the nurse said, "They are doing some procedures right now, so it will be a while, so why don't you just go on down to billing...."

In the end, the narrator's baby dies, with her teenage mother having had only one brief chance to hold her. Each request she makes to be involved in the care of her premature child is rejected because one member of the team or another is doing a "procedure."

Many studies suggest that physicians and nurses have a long history of communicating poorly with each other and failing to work as a team. Instead of a shared authority approach, a more paternalistic model has placed the physician in the role of leader, with all other health care workers subordinate to him or her. Studies suggest that this model leads to a higher rate of medical errors, especially medication errors. When a nurse is fearful of a physician (or other nurse), he or she is less likely to question orders that don't sound right, which leads to a higher incidence of medication errors—one of the leading hospital complications.

How RA Can Fracture a Functional Team

As you may have figured out by now, negativity breeds negativity. All it takes is one disruptive nurse to sour an entire unit. Not sure how your unit or organization rates? Look around and ask the following questions about your workplace:

- Do the nurses at my workplace frequently complain of somatic problems?

- Is our absenteeism rate higher than in other units?

- Is our turnover rate high? Do new nurses leave before completing orientation?

- Is there camaraderie among the nurses on the unit, or does everyone keep to him- or herself?

- Are we consistently short-staffed because nurses don't want to work on my unit?

- Are the nurses and other employees on my unit constantly unhappy and complaining about something or other?

- When nurses come to work each day, do they feel like they have to mentally prepare themselves for the shift ahead of them?

- Do I get subtle feedback from outsiders about the negative climate at my workplace (e.g., a physician who says, "Making rounds here is like getting through a minefield—I never know who's going to blow!")?

Much of the cohesiveness of a team depends on communication. As is obvious, RA is primarily a verbal behavior that can poison an entire work team. Even knowing that males and females come into work with different expectations can create issues at work and threaten the viability of a team.

Gender-Based Differences in Workplace Behaviors

Women	Men
Apologize for problems and mistakes, even if they didn't make them.	Fix the problem or try to find a definitive solution.
Want compliments and positive feedback.	Assume everything (including their work performance) is okay unless told otherwise.
Complain about relationships, sometimes as a way of understanding them better.	Loyalty prevents them from talking about others unless the problem is major.
Establish longer periods of eye contact when speaking.	Look away more frequently during conversations.
Interrupt during conversations.	Don't interrupt.

Women	Men
Self deprecate—e.g., "I look so fat in these pants."	Banter about others, but don't put themselves down in front of others.
Limit personal space in conflict.	Expand personal space in conflict.
Have relationship-oriented friendships.	Have activity-oriented friendships.

Creating a Unified Team

In the complex world of health care, it's hard to be a solo practitioner in any setting. Even if you aren't formally part of a team, at some point you'll have to communicate with others, if only to exchange information about a client or patient under your care. Okay—I just thought of a nurse I know who is a massage therapist. It's possible she will never have to talk to other practitioners, but most of us will.

Note that I said "talk" and "communicate." In this fast-paced world of 10- and 12-hour workdays, where charting is electronic and nurses call each other on cell phones, a lot of information gets passed around through technology. Taneva and Law (2007) note that "Clinical activity is not only a highly cooperative process, but also safety-critical, distributed over time and space, and characterized by high complexity and coordination demands" (pg.10).

If you or your coworkers are locked in a war of insults and other rude behaviors, the chance of errors increases while you're at work because emotions affect performance. If you go home and post something negative about your coworkers on your Facebook page, you've just quadrupled your chance of having problems when you get back to work. And if you fire off an e-mail to either the object of your anger or your nurse manager or supervisor, remember that these communications can not only be forwarded and shared, they can be printed out and become part of your employment record if someone is so inclined.

So what do you do if your place of work just can't seem to get it together? What happens if everyone can't leave their differences behind during the hours they work together? Hopefully, the person in charge will be smart enough to intervene and take action to promote a better sense of teamwork.

Relationships Are Everything

As positive, respectful relationships are promoted between team members so that every individual feels needed and important, the team will begin to coalesce. This includes from one nurse to another, one shift to another, and one hierarchy to another. Each person needs to matter in order to have the team matter, and the goals of everyone must be focused on patient care. Indeed, this is the goal of the entire organization—or it should be.

Ellingson (2002) says that health care teams can exist on a continuum, from virtually no interaction between members to highly integrated and mutually dependent interactions. Communication and diversity can be both an asset and a liability in health care teams. She believes that although there is always some conflict between team members, successful teams are a consequence of team members being able to sacrifice some autonomy in terms of roles and responsibilities.

Wilson et al. (2005) discuss high-reliability organizations (HROs) where high-reliability teams (HRTs) function within complex environments and are highly interdependent. These teams are committed to excellence, as demonstrated by their continued search for learning and new information, designing reward systems that emphasize the outcomes of both failures and successes, and stressing communication throughout the organization. The values of HROs and HRTs are shared: sensitivity to operations, emphasis on excellence, recognition of expertise, reluctance to simplify, and preoccupation with avoiding failure. Through these shared values, the team develops policies and procedures that circumvent error. Key to each is communication.

Relationships Are More Than Saying "Hi" in the Morning

Just as communication can be used for aggressive purposes, so too can it be used to achieve positive goals. Patterson et al. (2002) found that "strong relationships, careers, organizations, and communities all draw from the same source of power—the ability to talk openly about high-stakes, emotional, controversial topics" (pg. 7). They believe that when we find ourselves caught up in arguing, sniping, sarcasm, etc., we are usually operating from a position of fear or anxiety.

However, engaging in a meaningful dialogue with people you don't necessarily care for can be difficult and RA-provoking. Patterson and colleagues (2002) encourage asking oneself the following questions:

- What do you really want for yourself? Is being part of this team just a way to earn a paycheck, or do you really feel a need to cooperate in order to provide high quality patient care? Do you work best on your own, or in collaboration with others?

- What do you really want for others? Are the other nurses you work with just stepping-stones on the way to your success, or to you feel motivated to help them succeed, too? Are you proud of your coworkers' accomplishments, or does it secretly make you jealous when the spotlight is on anyone but you?

- What you really want for the relationship? Is the teamwork all about you and your needs, or do you see a bigger goal, and feel that you will sacrifice personal gains for the success of the team?

Just the Facts, Please

Just as assessing a patient's vital signs provides you with useful information about his or her health status, input from everyone on your unit or team is helpful in order to come up with a plan for change. Asking for employee input is a first signal that everyone counts equally—which is why you also want to collect data anonymously. Use the following questions to find out whether RA is destroying the team-ability of you and your coworkers.

RA and Team-Ability

1. Do you and your coworkers work as a team to achieve the same goals?

_____ Yes   _____ No

2. Do you think you play a role in promoting or detracting from the team spirit at your workplace?

_____ Yes   _____ No

3. If there was less relational aggression between the nurses you work with, would the sense of teamwork improve?

_____ Yes   _____ No

4. Is relational aggression a problem between the nurses on your shift?

_____ Yes   _____ No

5. Is relational aggression a problem between different shifts at your workplace?

_____ Yes   _____ No

6. Is relational aggression a problem between nursing administration and staff?

_____ Yes   _____ No

7. Using a scale of 1 to 10, with one being worst and 10 being best, rank the severity of the problems associated with relational aggression mentioned in questions 4–6

___RA among nurses

___RA among shifts

___RA among nursing administration and staff

8. Do you have coworkers you dislike so much, you just can't make an effort to get along with them?

_____ Yes   _____ No

9. Do you think your administrator/manager should be doing more to control RA within your workplace?

_____ Yes   _____ No

10. Compared to other places where you've worked, is there less teamwork at your current place of employment because of RA?

_____ Yes   _____ No

For a reproducible copy of these questions, see Appendix C, "RA and Team-Ability."

The E-R-I Approach

Whenever I conduct a workshop about relational aggression, I use the same Educate-Relate-Integrate (E-R-I) conceptual model as a basis for my curriculum, regardless of the age, profession, or any other attribute of participants. That doesn't mean I have adult women creating nametags with puffy paints and glitter—although during Club and Camp Ophelia Director Trainings, we do many of the activities girls will eventually carry out in the program. Sometimes trainees have so much fun, it's difficult to pry the glue guns out of their hands so we can progress to the next topic!

My approach is very systematic and based on the belief that you can't change a behavior you don't understand. For nurses who have had varying amounts of college work on psychology and experience with the human psyche, understanding the dynamics of RA can be a simple matter of awareness and education. For others, who may find themselves a little too uncomfortable with the dynamics described here, it can involve a more intense effort—repeated messages from different people and a persistent refusal to continue accepting what may be considered the status quo.

I suspect that's what was going on when I was asked to lead a series of miniworkshops for nurses on a unit where there were problems. Of course, seeing me and knowing what I'm going to talk about can be threatening right from the start, so I usually start with a story about girls because lots of nurses have daughters in the age range I work with. From there, I segue to my experience with adult women who continue with such behaviors—even nurses.

As I went through this standard introduction with my third group of nurses that day, nothing was happening. This was in contrast to my first two groups, who, by this same point in my talk, at least had a dialogue going. When I asked the first two groups why most nurses are motivated to go into nursing, almost everyone answered ("Caring," of course). Group three, however, was having none of it. They simply stared at me with blank faces, only occasionally nodding ever so slightly. Bravely, I continued on, describing RA and passing around an informational handout.

"So, what kinds of behaviors have you seen during your career as a nurse?" I asked brightly, careful to avoid any suggestion that there were problems right now on this particular unit.

One woman flipped her handout onto the table so that it spun away from her. "None," she retorted. "We don't have any of those problems on our unit, and we never have. I make sure of that."

Grateful for at least some response, I said, "Oh, great! So maybe we can talk about how you avoid RA."

Now she twisted around to look me in the eyes. "Are you kidding? I'm the nurse manager, and everybody does what I say."

I took a deep breath in. "Okay, well let's talk about some of the things that can happen when nurses *do* get into situations involving RA." Gamely, I continued on with my silent audience, who jumped to their feet the second I asked whether anyone had questions or comments (of course, no one did). On her way out, however, one of the nurses toward the end of the exit line leaned toward me long enough to whisper, "We have terrible problems with RA, but you probably guessed that."

RA Education

There are many formats to provide education about RA: all-day or one-hour real-time workshops, printed materials, conferences, staff meetings, and so on. Whatever venue you choose, remember that education is just the start—but it's often the most difficult step.

For example, admitting that you have engaged in RA behaviors—by gossiping more than you should—can be difficult. So can acknowledging that you suffer from the "disease to please" and go home depressed every night because you've allowed everyone to use you as their personal doormat at work, or even recognizing the many times you were a bystander who laughed instead of intervening as an aggressor erupted at another coworker. Typically, when I do an anonymous preprogram evaluation with girls, fewer than 5% see themselves as bullies. After going through Club or Camp Ophelia, that changes to anywhere from 20 to 50%.

For some, just knowing that what is happening to them has a name provides great relief. As I was working to make the deadline for this book, I received a long-distance phone call message from a woman I'll call Betsey. I confess I was typing furiously to finish on time and almost had my assistant tell Betsey to e-mail me, but for some reason, I called back. Betsey had gotten my name from the *American Journal of Nursing (AJN)* article I wrote on nurses and bullying, and wanted to talk to me because she thought I could help her. She went on to describe a situation in which her coworkers had clearly been relationally aggressive to her. Betsey loved nursing so much she had gone on to get a graduate degree, but at her workplace this was more of a liability than an asset. She also acknowledged that she was "fat" and that people didn't like that.

After giving her time to tell her story, I encouraged her to read some volumes listed in the Resources section of this book, and to understand that her coworkers were using behavior called relational aggression to break her down. (Given the fact that she was unable to get through the call without breaking down and crying, they appeared to have been successful.) Their verbal "slings and arrows" had nothing to do with who Betsey really was. But given the situation, it was easy to see how her self-esteem was below ground level. After encouraging her to find someone with whom she could continue the kind of dialogue we were having, we prepared to hang up.

"Thank you so much, Dr. Dellasega," she said before we ended the call. "I just knew if I could talk to you, you would be able to help me." I was glad she couldn't see how shamefaced I was for having almost not taken the opportunity to talk to her.

Relating RA to You

I have met a few women who say they have never experienced RA, but they do know what it is. In fact, the vast majority of women know exactly what I'm talking about when I mention RA. They remember the painful details around events that may have occurred decades ago. Most are victims, but a surprising number of aggressors have also come forward, expressing regret over the way they treated other girls in the past.

Even bystanders can have painful memories. Two women approached me after a lecture and described how they had watched as a classmate was systematically harassed, tormented, and threatened by another girl. The two women did nothing because they were afraid to get involved. One morning they learned that the aggression had become physical when the aggressor went to the victim's house and stabbed her to death. They vowed they would never watch violence and stay silent again. (As an aside, almost every physical act of violence between women is preceded by a prolonged period of relational aggression. Even adult women have confessed to striking out physically against a victim with whom they had an ongoing word war.)

Telling your story and being heard are also necessary components of the change process. The narratives in Appendix D, Scenarios, are true, with names and identifying details altered, of course. They can be used in a variety of ways to get a dialogue going. Reading a single story as a group and discussing the dynamics or picking out several stories and having individuals process them are two choices. You can also role-play the nurses depicted in the scenarios. My workshop evaluations tell me this is one of the most powerful techniques that help participants see what RA looks like and relate it to their own lives.

You can also convene a group as part of an RA workshop and have nurses write their own stories. If you choose this strategy, make sure everyone uses a plain index card and blue pen to write with so all examples look the same. Instruct the participants to leave out all identifying details, including their names or the names of other nurses. The purpose of writing the story is not to open up a gossip-fest, but to enable nurses to share experiences that have been difficult for them and obtain feedback from their colleagues.

Judy was surprised when she went through this exercise. "I had been good friends with Macy for a long time, so when an opening came up on our unit, I went to the nurse manager and suggested Macy for the job," said Judy. "Macy acted thrilled when I told her about it, but something didn't seem quite right. Macy interviewed for the job, but wasn't hired. My nurse manager told me that Macy wasn't qualified for the job, but I knew that couldn't be right—if anything, she was overqualified." She continued, "But then Macy stopped talking to me completely! Here I was, trying to do a favor for a friend and I end up looking bad in front of my unit manager *and* getting the cold shoulder from someone I liked. Macy and I never spoke again and my relationship with my nurse manager changed forever."

At the urging of the workshop group with whom Judy shared this story, she tracked down Macy, who had moved to another state. In a carefully worded e-mail, she asked if they could talk on the phone, and Macy agreed. "You wouldn't believe it," said Judy. "Macy told me my unit manager…called her in and asked a zillion critical questions about her work history, and then said she had heard Macy liked to date doctors! Of course, Macy assumed I was the source of that gossip. We ended up talking everything out and she apologized for thinking that my motives were anything but well-intentioned."

She also explained why she was now living closer to her family. She said, "Judy I didn't tell you but at the time my twin sister was going through a serious depression and had to be hospitalized, so I was upset anyway. I wish I had talked to you about what happened then and there."

So often, isolated incidents of RA are really much like Judy's situation. One person doesn't sleep well the night before, so she's a bear the next day, says something to a coworker she shouldn't, and a grudge forms that takes on a life of its own. So as you think of how RA relates to you, consider whether your coworker might be under stressors that make her act in ways she wouldn't normally.

Once you've figured out how RA relates to you, question how you've been affected by the events in your story or other incidents like them. Did you lose a friendship, like Judy and Macy? Are you afraid of confrontation because of an aggressor's past actions? Do headaches, fatigue, and stomachaches plague you when you're at work but mysteriously disappear during vacation?

Now It's Time to Integrate

Having educated yourself on what RA is and how it relates to you, the final step is to decide what changes you can realistically integrate to create a new relational you. Remember, you are a role model for other nurses. If you want younger nurses to have healthy and professional relationships with their coworkers and superiors, which of the following do you think is more likely to influence them: coworkers who engage in respectful but confident dialogue, or those who launch aggressive attacks that tear down their self-esteem?

One simple and relatively easy-to-make change is to focus on positive talk about yourself and others. Yes, it's a source of power when you know all the latest gossip and are the hub of the rumor mill on your unit. But sooner or later, relationships based only on what Club Ophelia girls call "trash talk" crumble and die. (After all, don't you encourage your daughter or other young women to avoid gossiping?) So the next time someone passes along a juicy bit of gossip, remind yourself of the four important questions about gossip, which you read about in Chapter 8:

- Do I know it's true?

- Will sharing it help someone?

- Would I share it if the subject of the gossip were here?

- What is my motivation?

I challenge you to start bringing out the best in the nurses you work with instead of obsessing over their flaws. In earlier chapters, you read about negativity fueling negativity; now you'll find the opposite is true. You can be the one who helps others have a vision, and every day someone can find your presence a blessing to them. I promise this will change your life, not just your career!

Exercise

Think about a relationally aggressive behavior that has been a problem for you or a coworker. Make a concrete plan to do something that will improve the situation around that behavior. Write it down and reread it regularly. If you want to really take the plunge, ask a partner to do this with you. Tell each other what change you want to make and how you plan to do it so you can hold each other accountable. Some ideas you might work on include:

- **Refusing to gossip:** When others start gossiping, you will walk away. If someone tries to tell you something directly, you'll say you can't listen just now.

- **Restoring a friendship:** Patch things up with someone with whom you've had a falling out. Tell her you're sorry about what happened and ask her to forgive you.

- **Using dialogue:** Use effective communication techniques when, say, discussing problems on the night shift with your supervisor.

10 | management mayhem: the role of those in charge

While individual nurses are accountable for their behavior and, as a whole, determine the reputation of the profession, much responsibility for their motivation and ability to function in positive or negative ways rests with the person who shapes their work life, be it a nurse manager, supervisor, CEO, CFO, or someone else. Laschinger (2010) says, "Creating a culture of respect in nursing work environments seems to be a point of leverage within nurse managers' control." Those individuals who control nurses' autonomy, their accountability, and what makes their job satisfaction high or low can do much to change the work environment by examining the degree to which RA has an impact on everyday work life.

However, Lewis (2006) notes that, ironically, nurse managers and their ilk are often on both the receiving and giving ends of RA. A study of 249 nurses in Washington State revealed that about a third had been bullied within the last six months. The biggest culprits were their nurse managers/ directors or charge nurses.

Eileen Dohman, vice president of nursing at Mary Washington Hospital in Fredericksburg, Virginia, believes that administrators are the ones responsible for creating an atmosphere where nurses thrive. She says, "My responsibility is the environment that nurses practice in…that's my job: To create, reinforce, and ensure that nurses have the environment they need to safely practice" (Hendren, 2011).

Unfortunately, due to the shortage of experienced nurses, many managers are promoted into such positions before they are ready to lead effectively. Rocker (2008) found that nurse managers often felt unprepared and inadequate when it came to dealing with bullying. She goes on to describe legislation that has been passed in Canada to deal with bullying, but says that most nurses are unaware of the laws. Instead, the expectation for a safe work environment falls on the shoulders of the nurse manager. She lists these interventions as possible ways a nurse manager can intervene to prevent or address bullying:

- **Education:** Help staff understand what bullying or RA is and what mechanisms are in place to deal with it. An outside evaluation of the educational program by an objective third party can ensure that the right information is presented in a non-judgmental fashion.

- **Policy:** Anti-abuse policies that address RA should be developed, with input from staff nurses. Including the suggestions and opinions of staff will underscore the seriousness of the manager's attempt to create a safe environment and signal her respect for those who work with her.

- **Recognition:** Include anti-bullying awareness and recognition of positive efforts and successes during nurses' week or bullying awareness week.

- **Diversity:** Leaders can be change agents, helping team members manage both perceived and actual diversity (Wolff et al., 2010) and highlighting shared goals.

When looking specifically at actions the nurse manager can take, Rocker (2008) suggests that administrators be very visible in anti-bullying efforts to underscore their commitment to ending bullying. Anonymous suggestion boxes and ombudspersons are other ways nurse managers can signal their interest in receiving feedback on how to improve the environment.

History of Past Problems

Most nurses are familiar with Post-Traumatic Stress Disorder and its consequences. On a more subtle level, Tobler and colleagues (2009) studied 19 healthy females and discovered that neural patterning actually occurs after repeated exposure to certain experiences. These changes lead people to infer probabilities from past experiences, with smaller likelihoods being overestimated and larger likelihoods underestimated. That means if someone was emotionally abused by peers in the past, they believe they will be emotionally abused again as an adult, even when they are in relatively safe positions and/or environments. Nurse managers in particular need to explore their pasts and look at RA experiences they have had—and at what impact those experiences might have had.

Grant (2007), a nurse administrator, shares the story of her childhood, when she was bullied so badly she developed a fear of confrontation that persisted into her adult years. Little did she know that when she accepted a management position, her confrontation avoidance led to an aggressiveness that became a way of life. Although she tried to learn healthy conflict-resolution skills, her behavior often veered into "self-sabotage," which involved taking out her frustrations on innocent bystanders. One evening, as she made rounds, a staff nurse made an inappropriate request of Ms. Grant, who writes:

My response to the nurse was abrupt and quite rude. I recall telling her that I was far too busy to carry out such a procedure, especially when they were obviously one of the best-staffed wards I had seen that day. By responding in such a short, blunt way, I then only provoked the nurse with an equally abrupt response… The conversation continued with this nurse stating she had heard how "intimidating" I could be and that I didn't intimidate her. I was extremely shocked by her response and ended the conversation by asking for her name and saying that I would be reporting her to her seniors. I left the ward that day shocked and deep down hurt by her accusation.

Although the situation was unpleasant, it also became a catalyst for Grant to do some self-assessment and reading. This led her to conclude she needed to change her interaction style. She says:

On reflection, this incident changed me for the better and made me take responsibility for my actions and response to others instead of using my position of authority. I began to take a step back when finding myself in similar situations, taking time to think of a response rather than answering quickly back in a negative manner.

How Managers Bully

Rocker (2008) suggests that nurse managers may have their own ways of aggressing against those underneath them which are variations of the behaviors nurses use against each other. These include behaviors such as the following (to name a few):

- Publicly disciplining nurses who have made mistakes

- Threatening consequences if nurses don't do what the manager wants

- Playing favorites

- Setting up certain workers to fail by withholding information

Stevens (2002) describes a hospital where a "bullying culture" was the reason for high turnover among nurses. In particular, during a series of focus groups, researchers discovered that staff nurses had been subjected to verbal harassment, exclusion from important meetings, criticism, and intimidation. One nurse claimed her entire unit was in therapy for work-related stress. The management style throughout all levels of the hospital was based on fear rather than respect. After an intensive effort to educate staff and increase the presence of senior administrators on the wards, the turnover rates declined by about 7%.

Stevens suggests that nurse managers can also undergo the same kind of healthy relationship training as individual nurses. Some components of this training would include the following:

- Improved communication
- Access to senior administration
- Policies specific to bullying
- Education on bullying/RA for all staff
- Conflict-resolution policies

He Said, She Said

With men being more likely to enter management positions than women (Lane, 1998), and male managers earning higher salaries than female managers (Hader, 2004), it's possible they may be the targets of RA regardless of how effectively (or ineffectively) they do their jobs. Gender-based differences in communication can influence work relationships as well. In her book *Talking from Nine to Five: Men and Women at Work*, sociolinguist Deborah Tannen notes that women who have positions of authority are less likely to use their power as a barrier between themselves and their subordinates, while men consider it important to appear in charge, with everything under control.

Hazel, a nurse who worked on a surgical unit, put it this way:

> *I was offered a promotion to unit manager, which I think I deserved since I had been there longer than anyone else and had the right credentials. My husband, Bob, and I talked about it and he was all for it since I'd be making quite a bit more money and working fewer weekends. But then I was like, wait a minute, I'm friends with all these nurses. If I become their boss they won't like me anymore. Bob just stared at me and said, "Are you crazy? You'll be making enough money to buy yourself some new friends. Who cares if your employees 'like' you?"*

Hazel ended up taking the job because Bob encouraged her to, but she was miserable having to discipline nurses she used to socialize with. Eventually, she transferred to another unit where she started over as a manager with nurses she didn't know, and her job satisfaction improved. Still, she was never quite sure she had made the right move, transitioning from staff to management.

Tannen (1994) observes how quick women are to apologize, even when they aren't especially contrite, believing that "I'm sorry" expresses more regret over what happened than an actual feeling of accountability for the problem. Men, on the other hand, are reticent to apologize, even when they are wrong.

Other differences Dr. Tannen found were that men intuitively knew that it was important to look good and get credit for accomplishments so they received good evaluations and promotions. On the other hand, women are information seekers. They like to ask questions and explore the answers. Although their motivation is to develop a richer understanding of the situation, their approach often makes them appear less confident.

Finally, Dr. Tannen describes differences in how men and women handle conflict at work. She describes men as being willing to give ultimatums or use other ways to pressure their colleagues into doing what they want. Women, on the other hand, engage in complex verbal negotiations to try to reason out the best course of action.

Of course, one could argue that men who enter the nursing profession are different from most and are more likely to communicate in ways that have been stereotyped as "female." It's also true that not all women and all men act in predictable ways. There are usually intragroup differences as well as intergroup differences. However, there appear to be no studies about differences between male and female managers, and since no nurses were forthcoming with insights, those answers are yet to be discovered.

Rx for RA

There are ways for nurse administrators to intervene on many levels to help employees conquer RA. Most involve following the Educate-Relate-Integrate (E-R-I) model used with individuals and described in the Stevens (2002) example in Chapter 9. But before taking action, it's necessary to know how severe the problem is. It's unrealistic to think that a group of nurses is going to sit down and talk about coworkers who are in the same room as them, so that means getting information in an anonymous way. Your goal should not be to identify a single bully, to punish problem employees, or to make examples of nurses who are stirring up trouble. But if your staff doesn't trust you, that's exactly what they'll think you're up to. When that happens, their willingness to give you any kind of information will be nil.

What options do you have to find out the "RA state of affairs" on your unit? Actually, there are several. One or all may work for you:

- **Use existing data:** Look at sick days, error rates, turnover, and the number of new hires who quit before completing orientation on your unit. Compare your unit to others in the hospital to see whether you are above or below average.

- **Hire an uninvolved third party to conduct focus groups with key informants from each shift:**

If you want richer data and a better idea of specific problems, you can look for an experienced focus-group facilitator who can meet with one or more small groups of employees and ask questions designed to capture the perceptions of nurses. It's crucial to hire an experienced person who knows how to create an environment of trust during the interviews and prepare the reports for you in a way that preserves confidentiality while accurately describing the nursing environment.

- **Administer a paper-and-pencil survey such as the one provided in Appendix E, "Survey of RA Work Environment":** Make sure respondents know that they don't have to complete the survey, but that if they don't, they will miss the opportunity to provide valuable input on their work environment. Obviously, the surveys should not ask for identifying information. You might even elect to use Survey Monkey (http://www.surveymonkey.com) or some other computerized form of data collection.

Once you understand the degree and types of problems on your unit, you can design interventions that will help to educate and change employees. Innovative strategies such as crucial conversations and the Conversations That Matter format espoused by The World Café (http://www.theworldcafe.com) can promote a healthy and informative dialogue that both educates and starts the change process in a safe environment.

Cleary, Hunt, and Horsfall (2010) suggest that managers can create a positive workplace culture by doing the following:

- Making sure everyone has access to the same information, as appropriate
- Asking for input and feedback on issues that affect individual nurses
- Avoiding authoritative directives, and instead offering explanations
- Not over-managing or supervising too closely (unless required)
- Being flexible in dealing with personal matters
- Being an advocate

Role Model

The nurse manager and the administrators above him or her truly are captains of the ship. As such, they set examples for nurses who work in their organization. Think of a nurse who was a positive role model for you during your formative years. How did she resolve conflicts, especially those situations that involved RA behaviors? Chances are, the reason this individual impressed you was because she had the ability to guide others without resorting to aggression and fear-based leadership.

If there are constant word wars between you and the higher-ups in your organization, it is inevitable that the front-line care providers will suffer from the fallout and turn on each other with the same kinds of negative behaviors. Although most nurse managers don't feel empowered to perform their jobs effectively (Regan & Rodriguez, 2011), they can be helped to change those attitudes. Communication skills that involve assertiveness without aggression can guide administrators at all levels to work more effectively with both higher level managers and front-line staff.

Exercise

Look at the list of RA behaviors in Appendix F, "Nurse-to-Nurse Bullying: The RN Way of RA," and add any others you can think of that are problems for the nurses you manage. Now create a list of behaviors that are the opposite (and therefore positive) of each RA behavior. Finally, list two strategies for achieving the positive behaviors. For example, if there is a lot of cliquish, excluding behavior taking place on your unit, how might you develop strategies so that no one feels left out and undervalued?

11 | the health care culture: in need of a cure

Felblinger (2008) reports that most Americans feel that incivility is a serious problem in our society. Additionally, 78% of those surveyed feel it has increased within the nursing profession—perhaps due to shortages and more pressure on nurses. In this study, 80 to 90% of health care workers report experiencing abuse, most often from physicians. Nurses are second-most common. (By now, I'm sure you've noticed that data fluctuates greatly from study to study, so it's difficult to know exactly what is happening in terms of who's bullying who, and how often.)

One disconcerting outcome is cited in a study that reported that more than half of nurses felt they had been subject to verbal abuse, while 90% had witnessed this behavior. The Institute for Safe Medication showed that almost half of the nurses said their relationships with co-workers interfered with medication administration because of this. That is, they were less likely to question a coworker perceived of as a bully—only one of the consequences.

On a personal level, nurses experience a shame response when these situations occur. They are often afraid to face their peers, who may agree with the aggressor/bully, and their self-esteem is lowered as they question why they have been chosen as a target. It also means the target keeps his or her guard up at all times, because the abuse may occur again at any moment. When you're spending your energy maintaining your defenses, it detracts from your focus on work.

Contagion

Organizational cynicism is a concept that suggests workers can become so jaded about their jobs that every aspect of the organization they work for seems negative. Although this outcome has not been explored among nurses, Volpe (2011) is one of the few researchers who has looked at professional cynicism among nurses and found a correlation between moral distress, job satisfaction, and cynicism. This means that feelings about one's job manifest in very obvious external behaviors, but the direction of the relationship is unclear.

Consider the Context

The overt stressors of working in the health care field are obvious: the sicker-and-quicker syndrome, chronic nursing shortages, information overload, and Internet-savvy patients. Yet we rarely think about stressors that occur on the most basic level.

Remember Maslow's hierarchy of needs (Huitt, 2007)? What other profession expects employees to go for hours without food, drink, or bathroom breaks? Where else are you "trapped" in a small space where it's impossible to avoid your aggressor? Sound pollution and excess stimulation is also a problem. What other environment is constantly noisy and constantly changing as physicians make rounds with their teams and patients come and go as quickly as possible? Going out for lunch to de-stress or having time to compose yourself away from an RA situation that has you ready to pop is a rare privilege for most nurses. Instead, RNs are expected to tolerate all of the above with a pleasant smile on their faces and a willingness to take on more if asked.

These factors are not excuses for shredding the self-esteem of your coworkers, but situations like Carla's are not difficult to understand. She described a recent 10-hour shift on her medical floor this way:

We were unexpectedly short-staffed because a new nurse had crumbled under the reality of long hours and the physical and mental stress of nursing and quit. Just up and walked off the floor in the middle of the morning. That meant divvying up her patients among the rest of us and doing the best we could until we got help. When doctors asked me questions about the new patients, I had to scramble to find answers, which made me look stupid.

I missed lunch, which is typical, but then a demanding family member of one of my patients got in my face because I hadn't answered his mother's call bell quickly enough. He even swore at me! I had to walk away because I was afraid he might hit me. So was I irritated when the second-shift nurse took her sweet time getting ready to sign on? You bet. I made a sarcastic comment to her about me working overtime because she took so long to settle in, and then snarled something like "Have fun" when I was finished. I'm sure she thought I was the world's biggest bitch because I felt like the world's biggest bitch.

Carla's coworker forgave her when she explained the situation and apologized the next day. Even so, knowing someone has the potential to launch a verbal grenade in your direction—even if he or she doesn't really mean it—erodes your trust and your perception of how safe you are emotionally when that person is present. And even though the other nurses who worked with Carla weren't targets of her anger, they saw what she was like when upset, and from that point on, their perceptions of her changed because they knew she had just as much potential to turn on them.

Other Kinds of Violence

McPaul and Lipscomb (2004) describe four typologies of violence in the health care workplace:

- **Type 1:** Criminal, such as robbery or theft
- **Type 2:** Customer/client, such as what happened to Carla when she was verbally harassed by a family member
- **Type 3:** Employee-to-employee
- **Type 4:** Domestic violence at the workplace

These researchers claim that nurses have very few options when it comes to modifying their environment, but draw on the Occupational Safety and Health Act to suggest organizational interventions. These interventions include the following:

- **Establishing a management committee for violence prevention and intervention:** The committee should be interdisciplinary, and responsible for addressing situations involving all four types of violence.

- **Worksite hazard assessment:** This focuses on behaviors to protect staff from violence. The quality and effectiveness of communication should be regularly evaluated as well as the physical environment.

- **Hazard prevention and control:** This is tailored to the facility. For example, an anonymous computerized reporting system could be used to identify employees who are chronic aggressors. Vanderbilt University Medical Center uses such a program to electronically monitor unprofessional behavior (http://www.mc.vanderbilt.edu/cppa). If a person's name appears repeatedly in the system, he or she is required to go through a special training on civility.

- **Training and education about violence:** This should occur at the time of hire and throughout employment.

Contrary to McPaul and Lipscomb's (2004) conclusion, however, nurses have more options for dealing with violence than ever before. The nursing shortage and high rates of turnover have made employers more willing than in the past to address concerns from nursing staff

(Knopper, 2009). Other factors that influence whether administration may be willing (or unwilling, as the case may be) to negotiate with nurses on work-climate issues include the following:

- The reputation of the institution

- Staff turnover

- Nursing shortages (or lack thereof)

Legal Aspects

Workplace bullying can be so devastating that victims often research whether a legal remedy exists. The answer, more often than not, is no. When bullying is motivated by age, gender, race, or disability, federal antidiscrimination laws may apply. Otherwise, there's no legislation to prevent one nurse from using subtle RA techniques against another. In a situation where, for example, one woman bullies another, or a female boss bullies a male underling (or vice versa), little can be done. Consequently, a victim of bullying who insists on taking legal action is usually limited to intentional torts, such as defamation (libel or slander), the intentional infliction of mental distress, or invasion of privacy. These actions are difficult to prove and unattractive to many lawyers.

Other Options for Action

Bullying in nursing has become so endemic that both the Center for American Nurses and the Joint Commission for Accreditation of Healthcare Organization (JCAHO) have released position statements urging zero tolerance for violence in the workplace. The Center for American Nurses says:

> *Lateral violence and bullying has been extensively reported and documented among health care professionals, with serious negative outcomes for registered nurses, their patients, and health care employees. These disruptive behaviors are toxic to the nursing profession and have a negative impact on retention of quality staff. Horizontal violence and bullying should never be considered normally related to socialization in nursing nor accepted in professional relationships. (Center for American Nurses, 2008, pg. 1)*

In addition to advocating a zero-tolerance policy for health care organizations, they list best-practice and evidence-based solutions such as the following:

- Working with other disciplines
- Education on effective communication
- Education and training about bullying
- Conflict resolution

- Empowerment of nurses
- Rewarding positive behaviors

Included in their statement are recommendations of specific actions that can be taken by individuals and on up to the organizational level.

The American Medical Association has also issued a statement on a model code of conduct, saying:

> *The AMA recognizes that "Personal conduct, whether verbal or physical, that negatively affects or that may potentially negatively affect patient care constitutes disruptive behavior. (This includes but is not limited to conduct that interferes with one's ability to work with other members of the health care team.)" (AMA, 2008)*

The AMA links bullying to staff turnover and quality of nursing care, and suggests that when nurses see such behaviors they feel insecure and unsafe. This makes the workplace an uneasy environment.

Researchers have shown how bullying work behavior can have serious outcomes, including the following (Knopper, 2009):

- Increased legal costs
- Threats to patient safety
- Increased medication errors

Usually, nurses are on the receiving end (50%) or at least witness it (90%). That's why the Joint Commission on Accreditation of Healthcare Organizations (JCAHO) required all hospitals to adopt a policy on bullying by January, 2009 (Knopper, 2009). In 2008, a lead news story outlined a new standard for hospitals by the Joint Commission, as of January 2009 (Aleccia, 2008).

The requirements arose from increasing evidence that bullying behaviors in the health care setting lead to multiple costly outcomes for both patients and coworkers. Hospitals are required to have a system to detect and respond to unprofessional behavior (EP4, "The hospital/organization has a code of conduct that defines acceptable and disruptive inappropriate behavior," and EP5, "Leaders create and implement a process for managing disruptive and inappropriate behaviors"). However, sexual harassment was not addressed, so the requirements lacked comprehensive coverage. Also, the notion of physicians being subjected to zero tolerance seems unrealistic. Are hospitals really going to implement consequences with any teeth in them?

Leaving Stereotypes Behind

In all the position statements reviewed, the issue of nurses aggressing against other nurses seems overlooked. The focus is on the physician-nurse dynamic. Discussions of the JCAHO standards relate in large part to the age-old stereotype of doctors mistreating nurses—which does still exist. But the sources reviewed for this book suggests that RN RA is the bigger problem.

Nurse-to-nurse conflict can occur throughout the 8 or 10 or 12 hours of a nurse's work shift, day after day. Confined physically to a fairly small workspace, it can be hard to escape your tormentor. It will be interesting to see what happens now that the problem of RA has been acknowledged and solutions are being sought.

Exercise

Think of a policy you might design to create a more civil work environment for your organization. What steps would be necessary for such a policy to address civility at all levels of the organization? How might you increase your chance of success? Consider options like Code Pink. With Code Pink, a nurse who is being harassed or bullied calls a number, and other nurses then come in to stand with her to act as a buffer against the bully. Another option to consider might be the Vanderbilt system of reporting offenders via computer.

12 | education, research, and clinical care

A multifaceted approach to change will involve nurses at all levels of education, research, and clinical care. The leaders in each field can be the ones to provide knowledge and certain kinds of expertise, but nurses on the front line are no less important.

Education

Randle (2003) found that students who witnessed other students and patients being bullied tended to internalize this behavior. In this way, RA and bullying became a "nursing norm," which led to low self-esteem.

This is unacceptable. Students at all levels need to learn what relational aggression is, why it occurs, and how to deal with it. Role-playing in the classroom can help provide practice for dealing with real-life situations, with classmates offering feedback (although a study by Cooper et al. [2009] discovered that 56% of students felt their classmates were the most frequent source of RA).

Each nursing program needs to have a strategy in place so students can report instructors or teachers who use RA behaviors or bully them in the classroom or clinical areas. Whether this information is obtained along with other anonymous teaching evaluations or in a separate survey, every student has the right to provide his or her input about teachers. Educators will take such feedback seriously if it becomes part of their yearly evaluation and factors into raises and promotions.

At the graduate and post-graduate levels, students should not be treated as faculty's servants and expected to perform additional work assignments for their thesis or dissertation supervisor. Again, a system for students to report abuses to the school's dean or director without retribution is also indicated.

Accrediting bodies should emphasize the importance of providing students—from the basic level on up—with valuable information about relational aggression. This material might be incorporated in a leadership or professionalism course, or it could be presented along with classes on effective communication or content on conflict resolution. More course materials such as podcasts, books, websites, workbooks, and other learning materials should be developed to supplement learning.

Nurse educators need to model healthy relationship skills and show respect for each other, even if they aren't particularly close outside the classroom. When on the clinical unit, teachers can show students how to interact with hospital staff in a way that avoids RA.

At the same time, when there are problems with RA behaviors, hospital administrators need to intervene promptly and work with their nurses. Seminars and workshops on healthy relationship skills should be presented regularly. Face-to-face meetings between hospital preceptors and nurse faculty who supervise students in clinical areas should also take place on a regular basis, whether it appears they are needed or not.

Research

Many questions remain about relational aggression and the nursing profession. First, a reliable and valid measurement tool that assesses the different domains and intensity of RA has not been developed, although my colleague Dr. Neil Montgomery and I are in the middle of validating a scale that examines relationally aggressive behaviors. Determining whether the aggression that occurs between nurses is the same dynamic as the aggression that occurs between physicians and nurses, nurses and medical students, or faculty members and students, will provide foundational data that will lead in other directions.

The gender issue is tantalizing. There is still a much smaller percentage of nurses who are male, so the question of bias is always present. However, understanding whether men take on RA as they assimilate into the nursing profession, comparing the types of aggression that occur between men and women, and studying relationships between males who are nurses with those who are doctors would provide valuable information about the origins and etiology of RA.

Different nursing specialties may also experience higher or lower levels of RA, as could different members of the health care team. "She thinks she's all that since she transferred to ICU," one nurse told me about a coworker who used to work on her rehabilitation floor. "Every time I see her she bugs me to put in for a transfer. She doesn't get it—I like what I do." Certainly, many nurses have told me they feel a certain arrogance from nurses who work in particular specialty units, giving rise to the "Supernurse" complex: nurses who can always perform better than everyone else, work with the most complex patients, and never be questioned about their abilities or actions.

Usually it's the "CUs"—ICU, CCU, NICU, PICU, and so on, but Trauma Services and EDs, as well as ORs, also seem to be accused of the same diva-like behavior.

Nurses who work outside the hospital report they have the lowest status of all. "Yeah, I can just hear it in their voices when I call," Maura, a home health nurse, says. "I had a patient in CHF who I got transferred to the hospital right away. While he was in transit, I called the nurses since he didn't have any family. The nurse who took my call kept sighing, and I could tell she was giving me about 10% of her attention."

The evaluation of promising programs and interventions should be undertaken as soon as possible. Is it enough to educate nurses on RA and hope they will change? Or is the entire E-R-I program needed? What other strategies have successfully turned units and organizations around and reduced RA? Best practices and evidence-based practice are perhaps the most pressing areas to pursue, because they can help stem the flow of nurses out of the profession.

Clinical Care

Reading the article "When the Nurse Is a Bully" by Teresa Brown, published on the *New York Times* website (http://www.nytimes.com), was an eye-opener for me. The number of comments from patients who felt they had been bullied by nurses was disheartening. And yet, it makes sense that if nurses on a particular unit are at each other's throats with hostility, patients will suffer.

As part of orientation, each new employee should be encouraged to report any problems with RA, and nurse preceptors should be taught how to precept. As one older nurse told me, "No one ever taught me how to be a preceptor. I just do what people did for me when I was young." Long-standing employees need to be educated about RA and reminded on a regular basis to avoid the behaviors. Whether that requires posters, fliers, a monitoring system, or some other form of surveillance that will keep the concept at the forefront of everyone's consciousness, it should be done. Organizational legislation and policies can back up efforts on the front line.

Keep Yourself Motivated

It's one thing to read a book or hear a talk and feel motivated to change. Actually trying that change out and then sticking with it takes a lot more effort. You'll be much more likely to be successful if you find some like-minded colleagues and tackle change as a group. There's no need to call yourselves something negative, like "The Bully Busters" or some other such thing. "The Self-Improvement Group" conveys the same idea. Hold each other accountable and set measurable goals that you can achieve on a daily and weekly basis.

Let's all work together so that instead of saying, "Nurses eat their young," the common wisdom will be, "Nurses know how to treat their young."

Exercise

Continue to journal about the changes you have been able to make and the feelings you have about your new behaviors. Note whether people react to you differently now that you're making a deliberate effort to communicate differently. Write a letter to a young nurse describing the lessons you've learned and give him or her suggestions on important "survival skills" for the first year of nursing practice.

A | RA quotient

1. I've changed jobs a lot because of the people I had to work with.

   _____ Yes   _____ No

2. I've left a job before my orientation period was finished because I knew I wouldn't get along with the nurses on the unit where I would be working.

   _____ Yes   _____ No

3. Every day, on my way to work, I feel myself becoming physically stressed because I don't want to go there.

   _____ Yes   _____ No

4. If another nurse does something rude or mean to me, I plan what I will say or do to get even with

her and strike when the opportunity presents it-self.

_____ Yes   _____ No

5. I'm always angry when I'm at work, but I rarely tell anyone.

_____ Yes   _____ No

6. I'm sick of watching the other people on my unit bicker.

_____ Yes   _____ No

7. People I work with don't like me, and I don't care. None of them are worth hanging around with anyway.

_____ Yes   _____ No

8. I take secret joy in seeing another coworker "get what she deserves" for poor performance.

_____ Yes   _____ No

9. My nurse manager/supervisor promotes relational aggression and bullying on our unit by playing favorites and creating drama.

_____ Yes   _____ No

10. Secretly, I think I am more competent than most of the people I work with. It's a shame.

_____ Yes   _____ No

11. Having good relationships among coworkers is important to the administration of my hospital/ organization.

_____ Yes   _____ No

12. I work harder than everyone else on my unit.

_____ Yes   _____ No

13. No one gets the last word with me. Even if I have to respond later, I'll make sure they know I can't be pushed around.

_____ Yes   _____ No

14. At least once a day when I'm at work I listen to gossip, pass on gossip, start gossip, or am the subject of gossip.

_____ Yes   _____ No

15. If I'm angry, I sometimes ignore or act rude to my coworkers as a stress reliever.

_____ Yes   _____ No

16. I get excluded from joining others in breaks or meals, or I do the excluding.

_____ Yes   _____ No

17. The emotional climate at my workplace is toxic because of the nurses who work there.

_____ Yes   _____ No

18. My feelings are often hurt by people/women I work with.

    _____ Yes   _____ No

19. I can't say no to my coworkers without worrying they will be upset with me.

    _____ Yes   _____ No

20. When I see other nurses being bullied, I feel bad. But I don't want to get involved so I say nothing.

    _____ Yes   _____ No

Add up the number of "Yes" scores you answered to obtain your score. The higher your score, the more RA you are involved in.

© *Cheryl Dellasega, 2006*

B | your RA inventory

Think about some of your interactions with other women over the last 24 hours and complete the chart on the next page. Look for themes in feelings or behaviors that suggest you might be in aggressor, victim, or bystander mode.

Your RA Inventory

The Place	The Person	The Behavior	What's Up With Me

Cheryl Dellasega, 2010

C | RA and team-ability

1. Do you and your coworkers work as a team to achieve the same goals?

    _____ Yes   _____ No

2. Do you think you play a role in promoting or detracting from the team spirit at your workplace?

    _____ Yes   _____ No

3. If there was less relational aggression between the nurses you work with, would the sense of teamwork improve?

    _____ Yes   _____ No

4. Is relational aggression a problem between the nurses on your shift?

    _____ Yes   _____ No

5. Is relational aggression a problem between different shifts at your workplace?

_____ Yes   _____ No

6. Is relational aggression a problem between nursing administration and staff?

_____ Yes   _____ No

7. Using a scale of 1 to 10, with one being worst and 10 being best, rank the severity of the problems associated with relational aggression mentioned in questions 4–6.

___RA among nurses

___RA among shifts

___RA among nursing administration and staff

8. Do you have coworkers you dislike so much, you just can't make an effort to get along with them?

_____ Yes   _____ No

9. Do you think your administrator/manager should be doing more to control RA within your workplace?

_____ Yes   _____ No

10. Compared to other places where you've worked, is there less teamwork at your current place of employment because of RA?

_____ Yes   _____ No

D | scenarios

The following narratives represent the types of stories nurses have shared with me over the years, either in person, via e-mail, or by writing. Names and details have been changed to protect identities. You can use the evaluation sheet provided to process the incident and come up with non-hurtful alternatives or as a prompt to discuss the scenarios as a group.

If you do choose to use the evaluation sheet, use the first column to identify the aggressor or bully if you can see one nurse who is obviously in that role. Be careful, though, since sometimes we assume certain people are using RA behaviors and judge them accordingly without having all the facts. The victim would be the target who got hurt (one or more persons), and the bystanders are those nurses who watched the incident occur. If you need to, you can consult the list of RA behaviors in Appendix E,

"Nurse-to-Nurse Bullying: The RN Way of RA." Most importantly, identify at least one alternative behavior that would not have involved relational aggression. This can help you begin to change the way you respond to conflict.

RA Scenario Evaluation

Marissa shared a story about her colleague Gail. "Gail came to me angry and with disappointment written across her face," said Marissa. "How could they do this, again? I had just learned the news myself: a job in administration had just been offered to Tina, the new girl, who had no experience." She continued, "The supervisors all agree Tina is 'very nice,' so that's why she got the job. Gail was denied a similar role a few years ago because she speaks her mind, defends her patients, and confronts adversity head on. Apparently, the focus was on 'nice,' the one word not listed in this job description." Marissa added, "The ongoing dilemma is which is more important—the ability or the agreeable personality?"

Aggressor(s)	Victim (s)	Bystander(s)	RA Behaviors	Alternatives

© *Cheryl Dellasega*

RA Scenario Evaluation

"My head nurse, Sandy, has a little clique going on," Mia said to me. "All the nurses want her attention, but she picks and chooses her favorites, taking breaks with them and even socializing with them." She continued, "I've never been one of her chosen because I won't do that kind of behavior. Not surprisingly, her gang usually gets the best assignments and opportunities." Then Mia brightened. "It's okay, though, because Sandy is just small potatoes when it comes to the nursing administration clique. I see her trying to use the same behaviors to curry favor with them, but so far it hasn't worked. She probably feels just like me—an outcast."

RA Scenario Evaluation

Anne, a nurse who worked in a community agency, recalled: "There was a new position in our agency and Beth applied. My friend Linda really wanted it, and because of longevity, she deserved it. Beth had her BSN, though, so they gave it to her." Anne went on, "We all decided to give Beth the cold shoulder and not help her out—why should we make life easier for someone who wasn't qualified and didn't have the first idea what to do?"

RA Scenario Evaluation

Rhianna published her first article, a small case study she thought was unique and interesting. Thrilled to see her name in print, she brought a copy of the journal to work and passed it around. Instead of the kudos she thought she might receive, her colleagues rolled their eyes and said, "So?" Later, Rhianna heard one of the other nurses talking in the lounge, describing her as "stuck up" and saying she thought she was so much better than everyone else.

E | survey of RA work environment

The purpose of this survey is to see how you feel about the emotional environment on your unit/workplace. Please do not put your name, anyone else's name, or include any identifying details in your answers to this survey.

RA stands for relational aggression, another name for female bullying, covert bullying, "drama," or word wars. It is nonphysical behavior that is used to hurt another person emotionally and occurs more often among women. Please give your opinion on the following questions.

1. Relational aggression (RA) and bullying are not problems for me at work.

   ____ Strongly Agree   ____ Agree
   ____ Not Sure   ____ Disagree
   ____ Strongly Disagree

2. My coworkers tell me they think RA is a problem at our workplace.

_____ Strongly Agree   _____ Agree
_____ Not Sure   _____ Disagree
_____ Strongly Disagree

3. Many of my coworkers are bullies.

_____ Strongly Agree   _____ Agree
_____ Not Sure   _____ Disagree
_____ Strongly Disagree

4. I wish someone would do something to stop the bullying and RA at my work.

_____ Strongly Agree   _____ Agree
_____ Not Sure   _____ Disagree
_____ Strongly Disagree

5. My job satisfaction is low because of the bullying at work.

_____ Strongly Agree   _____ Agree
_____ Not Sure   _____ Disagree
_____ Strongly Disagree

6. I would take another job if I had the opportunity because of the bullying at work.

____ Strongly Agree   ____ Agree
____ Not Sure   ____ Disagree
____ Strongly Disagree

7. My coworkers are good examples of supportive and helpful colleagues.

____ Strongly Agree   ____ Agree
____ Not Sure   ____ Disagree
____ Strongly Disagree

8. I have been a bully to other nurses.

____ Strongly Agree   ____ Agree
____ Not Sure   ____ Disagree
____ Strongly Disagree

9. I've watched my coworkers be bullied by other nurses and have felt uncomfortable, but have done nothing.

____ Strongly Agree   ____ Agree
____ Not Sure   ____ Disagree
____ Strongly Disagree

10. It's really true that "nurses eat their young" at our workplace.

   ____ Strongly Agree   ____ Agree
   ____ Not Sure   ____ Disagree
   ____ Strongly Disagree

11. Bullying and RA occur more often between older nurses.

   ____ Strongly Agree   ____ Agree
   ____ Not Sure   ____ Disagree
   ____ Strongly Disagree

12. Bullying and RA occur more often between nurses on different shifts.

   ____ Strongly Agree   ____ Agree
   ____ Not Sure   ____ Disagree
   ____ Strongly Disagree

13. Most of the nurse administrators are bullies and use RA to keep staff in line.

   ____ Strongly Agree   ____ Agree
   ____ Not Sure   ____ Disagree
   ____ Strongly Disagree

14. Male nurses are bullied more than female nurses.

_____ Strongly Agree   _____ Agree

_____ Not Sure   _____ Disagree

_____ Strongly Disagree

© *Cheryl Dellasega*

F | nurse-to-nurse bullying: the RN way of RA

Relational aggression (RA) is the use of a relationship to hurt others. Traditionally thought of as a female behavior, RA is sometimes called "drama," "covert bullying," "female bullying," and "catfighting." RA is not physical, like the kicks and punches of childhood aggression, so it can often be overlooked, disclaimed, or ignored by superiors who are in a position to help. In the hospital setting, it goes by many names: medical road rage, bullying, meanness, disruptive docs, nasty nurses, and so on. Some examples include the following:

- Giving another nurse "the silent treatment"
- Spreading rumors throughout the unit, hospital, or organization

- Humiliating or putting down another nurse, usually with regard to his or her nursing skills or abilities

- Failing to support another nurse because you don't like him or her (this could be anything from failing to help with care to disagreeing with decisions the nurse made)

- Failing to come to another nurse's assistance because you don't like him or her (a particular problem in EDs and psychiatric units)

- Refusing to share information with another nurse or otherwise setting him or her up for failure

- Excluding another nurse from on- or off-the-job socializing

- Repeating information shared by one nurse out of context so it reflects badly on him or her

- Running a smear campaign or otherwise trying to get others to turn against another nurse

- Sharing a confidence you were asked to keep private, and perhaps twisting it a bit out of context

- Making fun of another nurse's appearance, demeanor, or other trait

- Manipulating or intimidating another nurse into doing something for you

- Using body language (such as eye rolling or head tossing) to convey an unfavorable opinion of someone

- Saying something unfavorable, then pretending you were joking

- Name-calling

- Making a nurse look bad in front of patients, other nurses, or supervisors

- Teasing another nurse for her or his lack of skill or knowledge

The Joint Commission for Accreditation of Healthcare Organizations (JCAHO), which is responsible for regulating acute care organizations, takes this issue so seriously that as of January, 2009, they require policies to be in place that will help detect and address relationally aggressive behaviors. If your workplace has problems with RA, take some time to Educate, Relate, and Integrate:

- Educate by learning more about relational aggression.

- Relate the situation to yourself by examining your own behaviors on and off the job.

- Integrate by developing and carrying out a plan for healthier ways to interact with colleagues.

© *Cheryl Dellasega, 2008*

G | mean girls grown up: dealing with divas at home, work, and play

There are many words used to describe women who are relationally aggressive: mean girls, drama queens, queen bees, and worse. All refer to an *aggressor* or *bully* who is known for her ability to destroy other women without ever striking a physical blow. Instead, she uses relational aggression to humiliate, intimidate, and manipulate.

What Is Relational Aggression?

Relational aggression, or *RA*, consists of gossip, exclusion, teasing, tormenting, undermining, cyberslamming, and a host of other verbal and social behaviors designed to wound another person. Of course, men have been known to use RA, but they are more likely to be physically aggressive.

Who Else Is Involved?

Victims of RA are the targets of aggressive behavior, while *bystanders* are others who see what's going on and may or may not join in. In adult women, there seems to be less willingness to watch RA and do nothing about it. Bystanders tend to either join the attack in subtle or obvious ways, or walk away and distance themselves from it.

What Are the Consequences?

Believe it or not, adult women suffer from RA, which discredits the notion that "it's just a phase." In college dorms and sororities, girls report hostility, rivalry, and jealousy, especially when a romantic interest is involved. Later in life, the "PTO clique" can gain control of your child's school by allowing some moms to have power and denying it to others. At work, female bully bosses tend to be harder on other women than they are on men. Even within families, RA can ruin relationships and cause estrangements between mothers, daughters, in-laws, and ex-wives.

What Can I Do About It?

Lots! *Awareness* is the first step. Women rarely think of themselves as too aggressive, but in reality, every woman has the potential to use these behaviors (and probably has, on occasion). In the same way, each of us has probably been on the receiving end of a hurtful comment or part of the gossip conveyor belt.

But what if you don't exhibit any other kind of behavior? What if you're stuck in an *RA rut* without knowing it? If you feel constantly challenged by your female peers, take a hard look at your own behavior. Are you often the victim of attacks and put-downs, afraid to attract attention because it's likely to be negative? Or are you on the sidelines, all too willing to pass along a juicy tidbit of gossip when it comes your way? Could other women be alienated by your aggressive style of interaction?

Recognizing which role you play can be the first, but most important step in developing healthy relationship skills. Figuring out what might be motivating your behavior will reveal whether there are places or people that make you feel uncomfortable or threatened. Learning to communicate effectively, adjusting your attitude, collaborating around a common goal, managing stress, and sometimes just forgiving can help you end the RA way of life.

© Cheryl Dellasega, 2007

H | resources

Books

Ending Nurse-to-Nurse Hostility: Why Nurses Eat Their Young and Each Other by Kathleen Bartholomew (HCPro, Inc., 2006)

Researchers report that verbal abuse contributes up to 24% of staff turnover and 42% of nurse-administrator turnover. Additionally, studies show that approximately 60% of newly registered nurses leave their first position within six months because of some form of horizontal hostility. Bartholomew examines its many facets and offers strategies to make the workplace more peaceful and attractive to current staff and future employees.

Zapping Conflict in the Health Care Workplace by Judith Briles (Mile High Press, 2008)

Briles suggests how managers and staff can reduce and resolve conflict and sabotage in the workplace. She provides a detailed guide to awareness, prevention, resolution of conflict and sabotage, and, ultimately, the empowerment of all who work in health care.

Woman's Inhumanity to Woman by Phyllis Chesler (Lawrence Hill Books, 2009)

Chesler explores how and why women treat each other badly—what she calls the "shadow side of sisterhood." Based on interviews with women with horror stories, she urges all to break the cycle of cruelty among women.

Mean Girls Grown Up: Adult Women Who Are Still Queen Bees, Middle Bees, and Afraid-to-Bees by Cheryl Dellasega (Wiley, 2007)

Although primarily addressing victims of aggression by other women in the workplace, family, church, school, and even in feminist organizations, this book also advises aggressors and those who enable them. To help women overcome identified self-defeating patterns, the book recommends positive confrontation, working on self-awareness, and reaching out to other women for more satisfying relationships.

In the Company of Women: Indirect Aggression Among Women: Why We Hurt Each Other and How to Stop by Pat Heim, Susan Murphy, and Susan K. Galant (Tarcher, 2003)

Recognizing that a woman's worst enemies at work may be other women, the authors address differences between behaviors of women and men. They say that women should be more conscious of their reaction if other women try to undermine a promotion or honor coming their way. "That's the price we have to pay for the strong alliances we make with other women," they insist.

Mean Girls, Meaner Women: Understanding Why Women Backstab, Betray, and Trash-Talk Each Other and How to Heal by Erika Holiday and Joan Rosenberg (Orchid Press, 2009)

The authors look at hurtful behavior between women from the perspective of both the target and the victim. They use groundbreaking brain research to explain why being the target of a woman's hurtful behavior and being socially excluded can be so excruciatingly painful to women. Additionally, they offer compelling information for understanding the hidden dynamics (psychological, biological, and social, as well as media influences) that lead women to hurt or oppress other women and that compromise authentic female relationships.

Talking from 9 to 5: Women and Men at Work by Deborah Tannen (Harper Paperbacks, 1995)

A Georgetown University linguistics professor, Tannen looks at the differences in the ways in which men and women communicate in the workplace and how those differences appear to influence perceptions of worker skills and abilities.

That's Not What I Meant!: How Conversational Style Makes or Breaks Your Relations with Others by Deborah Tannen (Virago Press Ltd., 1992)

In this book, Tannen focuses on the uncomfortable moments when a conversation inexplicably breaks down, and suggests how such awkwardness can be avoided. She examines conversation style rather than psychological content and urges readers to look at ways to converse that either do or do not work for them.

Transforming Nurses' Stress and Anger: Steps Toward Healing, Third Edition by Sandra P. Thomas (Springer Publishing Co., 2008)

The nursing profession can't afford to lose practitioners to stress-related illnesses and burnout. Thomas tells nurses how to optimize their efficiency and relationships in the workplace, as well as how to solve work-related problems.

The book's third edition appeals to younger staff nurses and contains new research data, new vignettes from a variety of practice perspectives, current practice issues, and information on vertical career movement for staff nurses, managers, administrators, and educators.

The Twisted Sisterhood: Unraveling the Dark Legacy of Female Friendships by Kelly Valen (Ballantine Books, 2010)

Valen uses interviews with more than 3,000 women to demonstrate the paradox of how they both support and sabotage one another. Although the vast majority of women report having at least one female friendship they wouldn't want to live without, well over half said they approach female camaraderie with wariness or flat-out distrust, admitting that they are unable—or unwilling—to extend themselves to certain types of women. An overwhelming majority said they have endured serious, life-altering knocks from other females, and a solid 97% of those polled believed that improving the female culture in this country is crucial.

The Eight Essential Steps to Conflict Resolution by Dudley Weeks (Tarcher, 1994)

Weeks tells readers how to turn conflicts into lasting partnerships and ensure a fruitful outcome. Using his experience in conflict resolution, he says that problems that won't go away can be settled using methods he has developed.

Online Articles and Blogs

"When the Nurse Is a Bully" by Theresa Brown (http://well.blogs.nytimes.com/2010/02/11/when-the-nurse-is-a-bully)

Theresa Brown writes about the situation when a nurse is a bully and offers expert recommendations on what to do.

"Do Nurses Really Eat Their Young?" by Donna Cardillo (http://www.nurseweek.com/news/Features/05-01/DearDonna_01-10-05.asp)

Nurse Donna Cardillo tells why she's uncomfortable when she hears that nurses "eat their young," saying the problem is not as widespread as such generalizations suggest and ignores the many caring and collegial nurses working today.

"From Enemies to Friends" by T. Suzanne Eller (http://www.beliefnet.com/Inspiration/2004/02/From-Enemies-To-Friends.aspx?p=1)

This BeliefNet story demonstrates how a woman employee was able to win over an abusive male boss by deciding to be his friend.

"Horizontal Violence Among Nursing Students" by Joy Longo (http://www.psychiatricnursing.org/article/PIIS0883941707000325/fulltext)

In a research study, student nurses in the clinical setting reported experiencing horizontal violence or "nurses eating their young." The types of behaviors most frequently encountered were emotional and verbal attacks. Some students did not report incidences of horizontal violence to their instructors, so it is important that the faculty be cognizant that such behaviors can occur and establish open communication to assist students in dealing with such behaviors.

Free abstract is available here: http://www.psychiatric-nursing.org/article/S0883-9417%2807%2900032-5/abstract. Readers who are subscribers could then get the full article if they wished.

"Nursing Management and Aggression" by *Psychiatric Nursing* (http://www.nursingplanet.com/pn/nursing_management_aggression.html)

This article in the open-access journal *Psychiatric Nursing* explores nursing management of aggression.

"Why Nurses Eat Their Young" by *Reality RN* (http://www.realityrn.com/more-articles/nurse-relationships/why-nurses-eat-their-young%E2%80%A6/542)

In this article, *Reality RN* interviews author Kathleen Bartholomew on nurse bullying.

Search Results for "Bully" (http://allnurses.
com/gsearch.php?cx=partner-pub-
9350112648257122%3Avaz70l-mgo9&cof=DIV%
3Acacaca%3BBGC%3AF8F7F5%3BFORID%3A1
0&ie=UTF-8&as_q=bully&sa=Search#1334)

Search for "Bully" on AllNurses.com for extensive links to
blog entries on personal experiences with and solutions for
nurse-to-nurse bullying.

"From Enemies to Friends" by T. Suzanne Eller
(http://www.beliefnet.com/Inspiration/2004/02/
From-Enemies-To-Friends.aspx?p=1)

Nurse Laura Stokowski talks about bullying in nursing as a
matter of dignity and respect. (Note that a Medscape mem-
bership, which is free, is required to read this article.)

YouTube Videos

"Disruptive Behavior, Part 1: A Slap on the
Hand" (http://www.youtube.com/watch?v=Z8g_
fkQb2F8)

Nurses who are rude and disrespectful to coworkers put
their patients at risk. In this video, former nurse Jill Duncan
recalls watching a senior nurse bully a medical resident. She
explains why this behavior happens, and how to respond if
you're on the receiving end.

"Ending Nurse-to-Nurse Hostility: Raising Awareness Video #1" http://www.youtube.com/watch?v=SjSBGj-sOcw&feature=relatedhttp://www.youtube.com/watch?v=SjSBGj-sOcw&feature=related%29

Juice Inc. partner Brady Wilson describes the missing variable—the amount of interference experienced on the job—in looking at what constitutes high performance by nurses in the hospital setting.

http://www.youtube.com/watch?v=SjSBGj-sOcw&feature=related

The expression "nurses eat their young" has existed for many years in the nursing profession. In her book *Ending Nurse-to-Nurse Hostility*, Kathleen Bartholomew offered a look at the impact and solutions to horizontal violence. This training video explores possible solutions.

"Ending Nurse-to-Nurse Hostility: Why Nurses Eat Their Young (And Each Other)" (http://www.youtube.com/watch?v=1IGPE9IbRFY&feature=related)

Breaking a long tradition of silence about a major problem that affects every aspect of American health care, Kathleen Bartholomew delivers a keynote speech outlining the problem and her solutions. This is a short excerpt from the address, which urges practitioners to return to their units determined to address issues they've long avoided and start to create healthy work relationships.

"Horizontal Violence: Do Nurses Really Eat Their Young?" (http://www.youtube.com/watch?v=0Hwk4BH3_FU&feature=related)

A nurse describes results of a research study on horizontal violence in nursing.

"Nurses Who Eat Their Young" (http://www.youtube.com/watch?v=w-XL15eIqpI&feature=related)

Five nurses demonstrate what to do and what not to do to create positive workplace interactions.

"Responding to Disruptive Behaviors in Healthcare—Hope for the Future" (http://www.youtube.com/watch?v=PsvsPld8ZeU&feature=related)

Acclaimed experts in the fields of conflict engagement and mediation in health care, patient safety, nursing, and physician wellness gathered for the Emerging HealthCare Communities inaugural event, held in Northern California in January 2010. This video was filmed during the gathering as a core component of the Professional Conduct Toolkit, now available through the Department of Defense Patient Safety Program website. Experts include

Ila Rothschild, Esq., Special Counsel, the Joint Commission; Jeanne Floyd, PhD, RN; Kim Hissong, MD; and Robert Robson, MSc, MDCM, FRCP(C). For more information, visit http://www.ehcco.com

Organizations

AllNurses.com (http://allnurses.com/index.php)

This online community boasts nearly 50,000 nurses.

American Nurses Association
(http://www.nursingworld.org)

The website for the American Nurses Association contains links to articles and postings on bullying.

Dr. D and Me (http://www.cheryldellasega.com)

Professor, author, consultant, and lecturer Cheryl Dellasega helps girls and women turn conflict into connections in a variety of settings, including health care.

Hopelessly Human Productions
(http://hopelesslyhuman.ca)

Canadian nurses Linda Bridge and Kathy Knowles inspire nursing professionals to strengthen their self-respect.

Nursing Organization Links
(http://www.nurse.org/orgs.shtml)

This site contains online links to many clinical and other types of nursing organizations, nationally and internationally.

SEIU Nurse Alliance (http://www.seiu.org/division/healthcare/nurse-alliance)

This site contains links to Service Employees International Union resources on bullying.

Student Nurse Journey
(http://www.snjourney.com)

This organization aims to decrease the dropout rate of student nurses by giving them resources to help them through school, including dealing with bullying.

The Nurse Friendly (http://www.4nursing.com)

This site includes links to many online journal and other articles, including articles on nurse bullying.

I │ references

Aleccia, J. (2008). Hospital bullies take a toll on patient safety-health care. *MSNBC.* Retrieved April 11, 2011 from http://msnbc.msn.com/id/25594124/.

Almost, J., & Laschinger, H. K. S. (2002). Workplace empowerment, collaborative work relationships, and job strain in nurse practitioners. *Journal of the American Academy of Nurse Practitioners, 14,* 408-420.

Alspach, G. (2007). Critical care nurses: Are our intentions nice or nasty? *Critical Care Nurse, 27*(3), 10-14.

American Medical Association. (2008). *Model medical staff code of conduct.* Retrieved April 11, 2011 from http://www.ama-assn.org/ama1/pub/upload/mm/21/medicalstaffcodeofconduct.pdf

Ames, A., Adkins, S., Rutledge, D., Hughart, K., Greeno, S., Foss, J. et al. (1992). Assessing work retention issues. *Journal of Nursing Administration, 22*(4), 37-41.

Anderson, K. (n.d.). *Say it better.* Retrieved April 11, 2011 from http://www.sayitbetter.com/.

Barash, D.P., & Lipton, J.E. (2002). *Gender gap: The biology of male-female differences.* New Brunswick, NJ: Transaction Publishers.

Barash, D. P., & Webel, C.P. (2002). *Peace and conflict studies.* Thousand Oaks, CA: Sage Publications.

Berman, D. (2010, March 4). The evolving workforce: Women at work. *Spacecoast Business.* Retrieved April 11, 2011 from http://www.spacecoastbusiness.com/the-evolving-workforce-women-at-work/

Boudrias, J. S., Gaudreau, P., & Laschinger, H. K. S. (2004). Testing the structure of psychological empowerment: Does gender make a difference? *Educational and Psychological Measurement, 64(5),* 861-877.

Brezendine, L. (2006). *The Female Brain.* New York: Morgan Road Books.

Brown, T. (2010, February 11). When the nurse is a bully. *New York Times.* Retrieved April 11, 2011 from http://well.blogs.nytimes.com/2010/02/11/when-the-nurse-is-a-bully/

California Nurses Association. (n.d.). Safe RN to patient staffing ratios. Retrieved April 11, 2011 from http://www.nationalnursesunited.org/issues/entry/ratios

Campbell, A. (1993). *Men, women and aggression.* New York: Basic Books.

Center for American Nurses. (n.d.). *Lateral violence and bullying in the workplace: Position statement.* Retrieved April 11, 2011 from http://www.can.affiniscape.com/associations/9102/files/Position%20StatementLateral%20Violence%20and%20Bullying.pdf

Chandler, G. (1992). The source and process of empowerment. *Nursing Administration Quarterly, 16,* 65-71.

Childers, L. (2004, April 26). Bullybusters: Nurses in hostile work environments must take action against abusive colleagues. *Nurseweek.* Retrieved April 11, 2011, from www.nurseweek.com/news/features/04-04/bullies_print.html

Cooper, J. M., Walker, J. T., Winters, K., Williams, P. R., Askew, R., & Robinson, J. C. (2009). Nursing students' perceptions of bullying behaviours by classmates. *Issues In Educational Research, 19*(3). Retrieved April 11, 2011 from http://www.iier.org.au/iier19/cooper.html

Crawford., T. (2009). Male nurses experience more patient abuse: Study. *Workplace Violence News.* Retrieved April 11, 2011 from http://workplaceviolencenews.com/2009/04/16/male-nurses-experience-more-patient-abuse-study/

Dayton, K. (1999). Procedures. In A. M. Haddad & K. H. Brown (Eds.). *The arduous touch: Voices of women in health care.* West Lafayette, IN: NotaBell Books.

Dellasega, C. (2001). *Surviving Ophelia.* Cambridge, MA: Perseus.

Dellasega, C. (2005). *Mean Girls Grown Up.* Hoboken, NJ: J. Wiley & Sons.

Dunn, W. (1999). *Sensory Profile manual.* San Antonio, TX: Psychological Corporation.

Edwards, S.L., & O'Connell, C.F. (2007). Exploring bullying: Implications for nurse educators. *Nurse Education in Practice, 7*(1), 26-35.

Ellingson, L. (2002). Communication, collaboration, and teamwork among health care professionals. *Communication Research Trends, 21*(3).

Fanon, F. (1993). *The wretched of the earth.* New York: Grove Press.

Felblinger, D. M. (2009). Bullying, incivility, and disruptive behaviors in the healthcare setting: Identification, impact, and intervention. *Frontiers of Health Services Management, 25*(4), 13-23.

Fletcher, K. (2006). Beyond dualism: Leading out of oppression. *Nursing Forum, 41*(2), 50-59.

Flowers, D. L. (2004). Culturally competent nursing care. *Critical Care Nurse, 24*, 48-52.

Freire, P. (2000). *Pedagogy of the oppressed* (M. Bergman Ramos, Trans.). New York: Continuum International Publishing Group. (Original work published in 1970).

Gilligan, C. (1993). *In a different voice: Psychological theory and women's development.* Cambridge, MA: Harvard University Press.

Gordon, S. (2010). *When chicken soup isn't enough: Stories of nurses standing up for themselves, their patients, and their profession.* Ithaca, NY: ILR Press/Cornell University Press.

Griffin, M. (2004). Teaching cognitive rehearsal as a shield for lateral violence: An intervention for newly licensed nurses. *Journal of Continuing Education in Nursing, 35*(6), 257-263.

Hamlyn Young Books. (1979). *A collection of nursing stories: Hamlyn Anthologies.* Author.

Heim, P., Murphy, S., & Golant, S.K. (2003). *In the company of women: Indirect aggression among women—why we hurt each other and how to stop.* New York: Jeremy P Tarcher/Putnam.

Hendren, R. (2010, February 16). Nurse leaders' role in promoting autonomy and accountability. *Health-Leaders Media.* Retrieved April 11, 2011 from http://www.healthleadersmedia.com/content/NRS-246568/Nurse-Leaders-Role-in-Promoting-Autonomy-and-Accountability

Horsfall, J., Cleary, M., & Hunt, G. E. (2010). Why is better mental healthcare so elusive? *Perspectives in Psychiatric Care, 46*(4), 279-285.

Huitt, W. (2007). *Success in the Conceptual Age: Another paradigm shift.* Paper delivered at the 32nd Annual Meeting of the Georgia Educational Research Association, Savannah, GA, October 26. Retrieved April 11, 2011, from http://www.edpsycinteractive.org/papers/conceptual-age.pdf

Hutchinson, M., Vickers, M.H., Jackson, D., & Wilkes, L. (2005). I'm gonna do what I wanna do!: Organisational change as a legitimised vehicle for bullies. *Healthcare Management Review, 30*(4), 331-338.

Joint Commission. (2008, July 9). Behaviors that undermine a culture of safety. *Sentinel Event Alert, 40*, 1-3.

Kirkhorn, L-E.C., & Banasik, J.L. (2010). *Pathophysiology.* St. Louis, MO: Saunders Elsevier.

Kivimäki, M., Elovainio, M., & Vahtera, J. (2000). Workplace bullying and sickness absence in hospital staff. *Occupational & Environmental Medicine, 57*(10), 656-660.

Knopper, M. (2009, January 17). Trends: Putting a stop to medical road rage. *Workplace Bullying Institute.* Retrieved April 11, 2011 from http://www.workplacebullying.org/2009/01/17/trends-putting-a-stop-to-medical-road-rage/

Lane, N. (1998). Barriers to women's progression into nurse management in the National Health Service. *Women in Management Review, 13*(5), 184-191.

Leininger, M. (1991). *Culture care diversity and universality: A theory of nursing.* New York: National League for Nursing Press.

Lewis, M.A. (2006). Nurse bullying: Organizational considerations in the maintenance and perpetration of health care bullying cultures. *Journal of Nursing Management,* 14, 52-58. Retrieved April 11, 2011, from http://0-web.ebscohost.com.aupac.lib.athabascau.ca/ehost/pdf?vid=3&hid=22&sid=4d7ab594-a14d-4198-ad77-47da9c537cb0%40sessionmgr9

Linden, M. (2003). PTED: Post-traumatic embitterment disorder. *Psychotherapy & Psychomatics, 72*(4), 195-202.

Manderino, M.A., & Berkey, N. (1997). Verbal abuse of staff nurses by physicians. *Journal of Professional Nursing, 3*(1), 48-55.

Manojlovich, M. (2007, January 31). Power and empowerment in nursing: Looking backward to inform the future. *OJIN: The Online Journal of Issues in Nursing, 12*(1), Manuscript 1.

Manojlovich, M., & DeCicco, B. (2007). Healthy work environments: Nurse-physician communication, and patients' outcomes. *American Journal of Critical Care, 16,* 536-543.

McPhaul, K., & Lipscomb, J. (2004, September 30). Workplace violence in health care: Recognized but not regulated. *Online Journal of Issues in Nursing, 9*(3), Manuscript 6. Retrieved April 11, 2011from www.nursingworld.org/MainMenuCategories/ANAMarketplace/ANAPeriodicals/OJIN/TableofContents/Volume92004/No3Sept04/ViolenceinHealthCare.aspx

O'Lynn, C. E., & Tranbarger, R. E. (Eds.) (2006). *Men in nursing: History, challenges, and opportunities*. New York: Springer Pub.

Parsons, M. L., & Stonestreet, J. (2004). Staff nurse retention: Laying in groundwork by listening. *Nursing Leadership Forum, 8*(3), 107-113.

Patterson, K., Grenny, J., McMillan, R., Switzler, A., & Covey, S. (2002). *Crucial conversations: Tools for talking when stakes are high*. New York: McGraw-Hill.

Pipher, M. B. (1994). *Reviving Ophelia: Saving the selves of adolescent girls*. New York: Putnam.

Quine, L. (2001). Workplace bullying in nurses. *Journal of Health Psychology, 6*, 73-84.

Ramsey, G. (1997). A glass of milk in the night. In B. Finkelstein (Ed.), *My first year as a nurse: Real-world stories from America's nurses*. New York: Signet Books.

Randle, J. (2003). Changes in self-esteem during a 3-year pre-registration Diploma in Higher Education (Nursing) programme. *Journal of Clinical Nursing, 12*(1), 142-143.

Regan, L. C., & Rodriguez, L. (2011). Nurse empowerment from a middle-management perspective: Nurse managers' and assistant nurse managers' workplace empowerment views. *The Permanente Journal, 15*(1).

Rocker, C. (2008, August 29). Addressing nurse-to-nurse bullying to promote nurse retention. *OJIN: The Online Journal of Issues in Nursing, 13*(3).

Rosenstein, A.H., & O'Daniel, M. (2005). Disruptive behavior and clinical outcomes: Perceptions of nurses and physicians. *American Journal of Nursing, 105*(1), 26-34.

Shader, K., Broome, M.E., West, M.E. & Nash, M. (2001). Factors influencing satisfaction and anticipated turnover for nurses in an academic medical center. *Journal of Nursing Administration, 31*, 210-216.

Songer, E. (2007, October 10). Top ten reasons I love being a registered nurse. Associated Content from YAHOO! Retrieved April 11, 2011 from http://www.associatedcontent.com/article/399286/top_ten_reasons

Stevens, S. (2002). Nursing workforce retention: Challenging a bullying culture. *Health Affairs, 21*(5), 189–193.

Stringer, H. (2001, February 12). Raging bullies: A disturbing number of nurses face verbal abuse, mostly from physicians, and some hospitals are taking steps to improve relations. *NurseWeek*. Retrieved April 11, 2011 from http://www.nurseweek.com/news/features/01-02/bully.asp

Taber's Cyclopedic Medical Dictionary. (n.d.). *Caring behaviors*. Retrieved April 11, 2011 from http://www.tabers.com/tabersonline/ub/view/Tabers/143111/47/caring_behaviors?q=caring behaviors

Taneva, S., & Law, E. (2007). *Interfacing safety and communication breakdowns: Situated medical technology design*. Proceedings of the 12th International Conference on Human Computer Interaction, Beijing, China.

Tannen, D. (1994). *Talking from 9 to 5: How women's and men's conversational styles affect who gets heard, who gets credit, and what gets done at work*. New York: William Morrow and Company.

Taylor, S.E. (2002). *The tending instinct: How nurturing is essential for who we are and how we live*. New York: Times Books.

Tobler, P.N., Christopoulos, G.I., O'Doherty, J.P., Dolan, R.J., & Schultz, W. (2009, April 28). Risk-dependent reward value signal in human prefrontal cortex. Proceedings of the National Academy of Sciences of the United States of America, *106*, 7185-7190.

U.S. Department of Health and Human Services. (2010). *The registered nurse population: Findings from the 2008 National Sample Survey of Registered Nurses.* Retrieved April 11, 2011 from http://bhpr.hrsa.gov/healthworkforce/rnsurvey/2008/nssrn2008.pdf

U.S. Department of Labor. (2009, January). *Employment & earnings, 56*(1). Retrieved April 11, 2011 from http://www.bls.gov/opub/ee/empearn200901.pdf

Ulrich, B.T, Lavandero, R., Hart, K.A., Woods, D., Leggett, J., & Taylor, D. (2006). Critical care nurses' work environments: A baseline status report. *Critical Care Nurse, 26,* 46-57.

Vance. T. (n.d.). Caring and the professional practice of nursing. *RN Journal.* Retrieved April 11, 2011 from http://www.rnjournal.com/journal_of_nursing/caring.htm

Vessey, J., Demarco, R., Gaffney, D., & Budin, W. (2009). Bullying of staff registered nurses in the workplace: A preliminary study for developing personal and organizational strategies for the transformation of hostile to healthy workplace environments. *Journal of Professional Nursing, 25*(5), 299-306.

Wilson, K. A., Burke, C. S., Priest, H., & Salas, E. (2005). Promoting health care safety through training high reliability teams. *Quality and Safety in Health Care, 14,* 303-309.

Wolf, N. (1990). *The beauty myth*. New York: W. Morrow.

Wolff, A.C., Ratner, P.A., Robinson, S.L., Oliffe, J.L., & Hall, L.M. (2010). Beyond generational differences: A literature review of the impact of relational diversity on nurses' attitudes and work. *Journal of Nursing Management, 18*, 948-969.

Wuest, J. (1994). Professionalism and the evolution of nursing as a discipline: A feminist perspective. *Journal of Professional Nursing, 10*(6), 357-367.

index